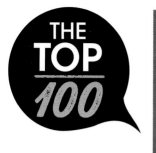

THE TOP 100 / 100

Low Carb Recipes

D0263304

523 386 69 0

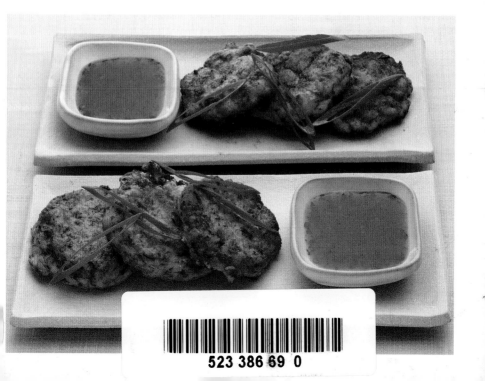

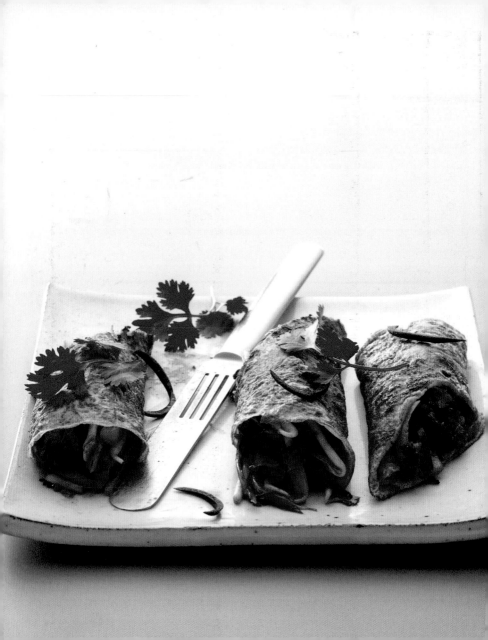

Nicola Graimes

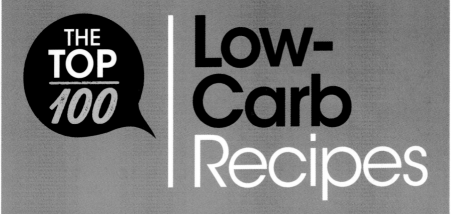

THE
TOP
100

Low-
Carb
Recipes

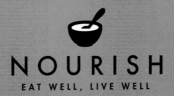

NOURISH
EAT WELL, LIVE WELL

First published in the UK and USA in 2016 by
Nourish, an imprint of Watkins Media Limited
19 Cecil Court, London WC2N 4EZ

enquiries@nourishbooks.com

Recipes taken from *The Big Book of Low-Carb
Recipes*, first published by DBP in 2005

Managing Editor: Sarah Epton
Designer: Clare Thorpe
Commissioned photography: William Lingwood
Photography Assistant: Estelle Cuthbert
Food Stylist: David Morgan
Prop Stylist: Helen Trent

A CIP record for this book is available from the
British Library

ISBN: 978-1-84899-302-0

10 9 8 7 6 5 4 3 2 1

Typeset in Avant Garde Gothic
Colour reproduction by Scanhouse, Malaysia
Printed in China

Publisher's note

While every care has been taken in compiling
the recipes for this book, Watkins Media
Limited, or any other persons who have been
involved in working on this publication, cannot
accept responsibility for any errors or omissions,
inadvertent or not, that may be found in the
recipes or text, nor for any problems that may
arise as a result of preparing one of these recipes.
If you are pregnant or breastfeeding or have
any special dietary requirements or medical
conditions, it is advisable to consult a medical
professional before following any of the recipes
contained in this book.

Notes on the recipes

Unless otherwise stated:
Use free-range or organic eggs
Use medium fruit and vegetables
Use fresh ingredients, including herbs and spices
Do not mix metric and imperial measurements
1 tsp = 5ml / $\frac{1}{8}$fl oz
1 tbsp = 15ml / $\frac{1}{2}$fl oz
1 cup = 240ml / 8fl oz

nourishbooks.com

CONTENTS

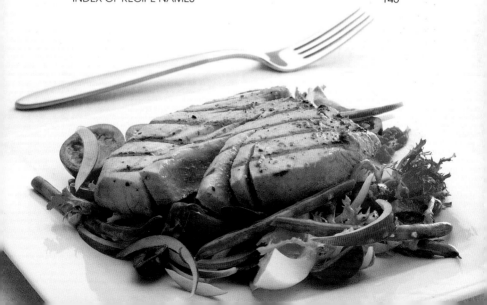

INTRODUCTION

Carbohydrates are an essential part of our diet and a primary source of energy. However, there are different types of carbohydrates and each has a differing effect on blood glucose and insulin levels, which in turn affect how we feel. Controlling the effects of carbohydrates in the body is important if you want to lose weight and maintain a healthy weight in the long term without being left feeling hungry, frustrated and miserable. The nutritious recipes here offer ideas for using so-called 'good carbs' and carbs with a low glycaemic index, while cutting out refined and processed foods that help pile on the weight. Healthy eating should always be combined with exercise and drinking enough water – both vital for good health.

CARBOHYDRATES – THE 'GOOD' AND 'BAD' GUYS

There are certain carbs that play no role in our diet and are basically nutritionally redundant. These are the refined types, such as sugar and white flour, which during processing are stripped of their fibre content and of many of their nutrients. 'Bad' carbohydrates also influence blood glucose and insulin levels, resulting in peaks and troughs in energy levels, cravings for more carbohydrates and hunger pangs. Foods made up of refined flour and sugar also tend to contain significant amounts of fat, responsible for adding excess weight. The following foods are our most familiar 'bad' carbohydrates:

• white pasta and rice • white bread • refined sugar • biscuits/cookies and cakes • chocolate and sweets/candy • crisps/potato chips and salted nuts • sugary breakfast cereals and cereal bars • fizzy drinks/sodas, cordials and juice drinks • pre-packaged convenience meals • pizzas and pies • ready-made sauces and gravy mixes

By contrast, the 'good' carbs (for example, wholemeal/whole-wheat pasta, pulses, whole grain bread and brown rice) provide valuable vitamins and minerals as well as fibre. By eating these in controlled amounts and in combination with other food groups, you'll avoid highs and lows in blood glucose levels that result in dramatic energy fluctuations and hunger pangs.

WHAT YOU NEED EVERY DAY

A carbohydrate intake of around 40 per cent of your daily calorie intake is recommended, but this varies from person to person depending on activity levels and metabolism. When deciding which carbs to include in your diet, avoid overloading on wheat as the easy option. Try other types of grain, such as oats, barley or rye, and for gluten-free alternatives try quinoa, buckwheat or rice.

Regular meals based on the main food groups ('good' carbs, lean protein, healthy fats, and plenty of vegetables) help to control appetite and how we store fat in the body. Many diets suggest cutting carbs out of the evening meal, but they do have an influence on serotonin levels in the brain and consequently on how we sleep, so it is advisable to include some form of unrefined carbohydrate in tandem with protein in your last meal of the day.

ABOUT THE RECIPES IN THIS BOOK

Each person's tolerance to carbohydrates is different. This is why at the end of each recipe you will find an approximate carb count, which enables you to choose and balance the dishes depending on whether you are looking to lose weight or maintain a healthy weight level.

The recipes have been created to fit in with our fast-paced lives; they're simple and in the main quick to prepare, making the most of fresh, quality ingredients from many cuisines around the world.

Chapter One

Breakfasts & Brunches

Breakfast is traditionally high in carbohydrates but it doesn't have to be, as the varied selection of recipes in this chapter demonstrates. Whether you're looking for ideas for a quick weekday breakfast or a more leisurely weekend brunch, there's a recipe for you. It's tempting to skip breakfast when weight loss is an issue, but research has shown that cutting what is often considered to be the most important meal of the day can lead to an undesirable pattern of snacking on unhealthy foods mid-morning. We need to eat a good breakfast to replace some of the glycogen stores diminished overnight, to refuel the body with essential nutrients and to provide energy for the morning ahead. Protein foods, such as lean meat, poultry, fish, tofu, eggs, nuts and seeds rapidly satiate the appetite for long periods, keeping hunger pangs at bay. However, don't forget your good carbs, particularly those with a low glycaemic index value, as these will help to keep blood sugar levels steady, providing much-needed sustained energy as well as fibre. The following breakfast recipes have all been selected bearing these dietary considerations in mind and the emphasis is on taste, variety and health, rather than deprivation.

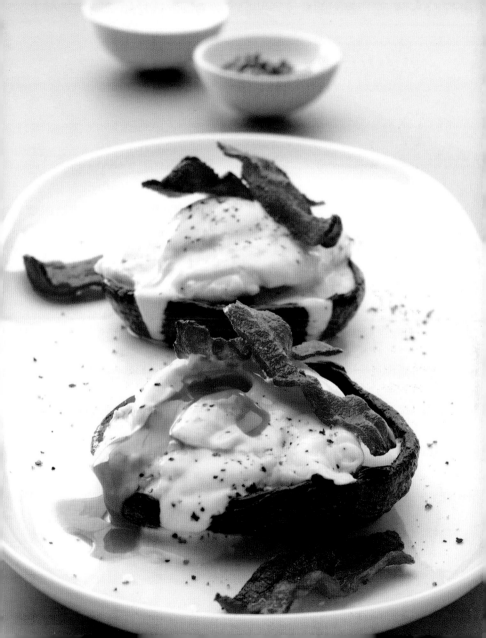

001

ROASTED MUSHROOMS WITH CRÈME FRAÎCHE & BACON SERVES 2

2 large portobello mushrooms
1 tbsp extra-virgin olive oil
2 eggs

2 tbsp reduced-fat crème fraîche
2 slices bacon, grilled/broiled until crisp
salt and freshly ground black pepper

1   Preheat the oven to 200°C/400°F/Gas 6. Place the mushrooms in a piece of foil large enough to make a parcel. Spoon over the oil and season. Fold up the foil to encase the mushrooms. Place the parcel on a baking sheet and roast for 20 minutes until tender.

2   Meanwhile, half-fill a frying pan with water and bring to a boil, then reduce the heat to low. Break the eggs into the pan and cook them at a gentle simmer for about 3 minutes, then remove using a slotted spoon and drain.

3   Place a mushroom on each serving plate and top with a poached egg. Place a spoonful of crème fraîche on top of each one and sprinkle with the bacon snipped into small pieces. Season with salt and pepper.

3G CARBOHYDRATE PER SERVING

BREAKFASTS & BRUNCHES

Recipe pictured on page 9

002

SMOKED SALMON OMELETTE

SERVES 1

small knob of butter
2 eggs, beaten
few strips smoked salmon
freshly ground black pepper

extra-virgin olive oil, for brushing
2 vine-ripened tomatoes, thickly sliced
$\frac{1}{2}$ tsp balsamic vinegar (optional)

1   Melt the butter in a medium-size frying pan and swirl it around to coat the bottom.
2   Pour in the egg and as it sets, gently push the edges towards the middle, allowing
    the raw egg to run to the edges of the pan. Place the salmon in the middle then
    cook until the egg is lightly set but still runny on top.
3   Season the omelette with pepper, then fold in half to enclose the salmon and
    heat briefly.
4   Meanwhile, heat a grill/broiler to medium. Line a grill/broiler pan with foil and
    brush with a little olive oil. Arrange the tomato slices on top and grill/broil for about
    3 minutes, turning, until tender.
5   Place the omelette and grilled/broiled tomatoes on a plate. Spoon the balsamic
    vinegar over the tomatoes, if using.

2.5G CARBOHYDRATE PER SERVING

003

SUNDAY BREAKFAST PLATTER

SERVES 2

4 slices prosciutto
1 hard-boiled egg, quartered
55g/2oz Gruyère, thinly sliced
6 spears of asparagus, trimmed and
  steamed
2 small slices rye bread

RICOTTA DIP:
5 tbsp ricotta cheese
2 tbsp snipped fresh chives
1 tbsp chopped fresh basil
1 tbsp lemon juice
salt and freshly ground black pepper
paprika, to garnish

1   Arrange the prosciutto, egg, Gruyère, asparagus and rye bread on a serving
    platter.
2   Put the ricotta, chives, basil and lemon juice in a blender. Process until creamy.
    Season to taste and spoon into a small serving bowl. Sprinkle with paprika to serve.

15G CARBOHYDRATE PER SERVING

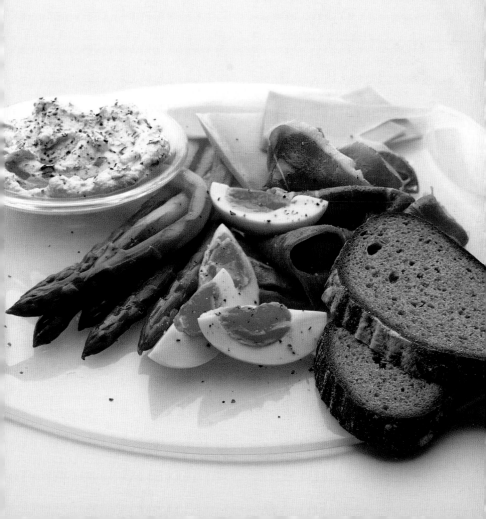

004

BREAKFAST FRITTATA SERVES 4

4 good-quality gluten-free sausages
  (or vegetarian alternative)
olive oil, for frying

12 cherry tomatoes
6 eggs, beaten
salt and freshly ground black pepper

1   Preheat the grill/broiler to medium-high. Arrange the sausages on a foil-lined
    grill/broiler pan and cook until golden. Leave to cool slightly, then slice into
    bite-size pieces.

2   Meanwhile, heat a little oil in a medium-size frying pan with a heatproof handle,
    add the tomatoes and cook for 2 minutes. Arrange the sausages in the pan so the
    tomatoes and sausages are evenly distributed.

3   Add a little more oil to the pan if it seems dry. Season the beaten eggs and pour
    the mixture over the ingredients in the pan. Cook for 5 minutes without stirring
    the omelette, until the base is set and light golden. Place the pan under the
    preheated grill/broiler for an additional 3 minutes until the top is just cooked.
    Serve cut into wedges.

4G CARBOHYDRATE PER SERVING

005

EGGS FLORENTINE SERVES 2

250g/9oz/4½ cups baby spinach leaves, rinsed well

3 tbsp reduced-fat crème fraîche

a little grated nutmeg

2 large eggs

40g/1½oz/⅓ cup grated mature Cheddar

salt and freshly ground black pepper

1 Steam the spinach for 2 minutes until wilted. Leave to drain, then squeeze out any excess water using your hands. Finely chop the spinach, then mix with the crème fraîche and a little grated nutmeg. Season and spoon the spinach mixture into a small baking dish.

2 Preheat the grill/broiler to medium. Make two hollows in the spinach mixture, large enough to accommodate the eggs. Break the eggs into the holes, top the eggs with cheese and grill/broil for 2–3 minutes until the eggs are just set.

3G CARBOHYDRATE PER SERVING

BREAKFASTS & BRUNCHES

006

TORTILLA EGG ROLLS SERVES 2

2 small wholemeal/whole-wheat flour
   tortillas or pitta breads
8 vine-ripened cherry tomatoes, grilled/
   broiled, or oven-baked, to serve

FILLING:
15g/½oz/1 tbsp unsalted butter
1 tsp olive oil

¼ red pepper, seeded and diced
1 spring onion/scallion, finely chopped
2 sun-dried tomatoes in oil, drained and
   finely chopped
4 eggs, lightly beaten
2 tbsp milk
salt and freshly ground black pepper

1   To make the filling, heat the butter and oil in a heavy saucepan, add the
    pepper, spring onion/scallion and sun-dried tomatoes and cook for 5 minutes
    until softened.

2   Mix together the eggs and milk, season well, then pour into the pan. Using a
    wooden spoon, stir the egg constantly but gently, to ensure it doesn't stick.
    Cook for about 2–3 minutes until the scrambled egg is semi-solid but creamy.

3   Meanwhile, warm the tortillas in an oven or dry frying pan, then spoon the egg
    on top and roll up. Serve with the grilled/broiled tomatoes.

18G CARBOHYDRATE PER SERVING

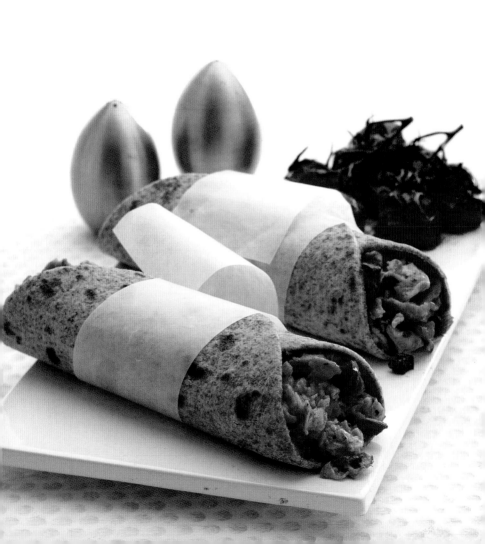

007

SOUFFLÉ BERRY OMELETTE SERVES 1

2 eggs, separated
¼ tsp ground cinnamon

small knob of butter
100g/3½oz/¾ cup frozen mixed berries, defrosted

1   Whisk the egg whites in a large, grease-free bowl until they form stiff peaks. Beat the egg yolks, then carefully fold into the egg whites with the cinnamon using a metal spoon.
2   Gently melt the butter in a medium-size heavy frying pan and swirl it around to cover the base. Spoon in the whisked, frothy egg mixture and gently flatten it (without losing too much air) using a spatula until it covers the base of the pan. Cook over a medium heat for 1 minute.
3   Spoon the berries down the middle of the omelette and cook for another 2 minutes or until the bottom of the omelette is set and golden. Fold the omelette in half to encase the berries and slide onto a plate to serve.

12G CARBOHYDRATE PER SERVING

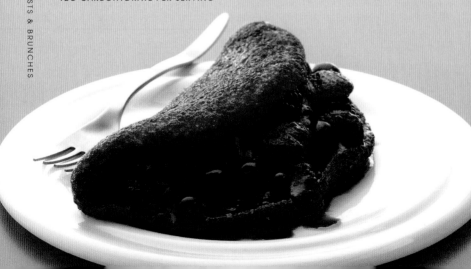

008

RASPBERRY OAT CRUNCH SERVES 2

1 tbsp sunflower seeds

1 tbsp chopped walnuts

200g/7oz/1 cup thick natural bio yogurt

1 tbsp ground flaxseeds

115g/4oz/scant 1 cup raspberries, fresh or frozen and defrosted

1   Place the sunflower seeds and walnuts in a dry frying pan and cook over a medium heat for 1–2 minutes until lightly toasted and golden in colour (take care – they can easily burn). Leave to cool.

2   Spoon the yogurt into a large bowl and stir in the flaxseeds.

3   If using frozen raspberries, allow them to defrost. Gently fold the raspberries into the yogurt and stir to give a marbled effect. Spoon into 2 glasses and top with the toasted seeds and nuts before serving.

16G CARBOHYDRATE PER SERVING

Chapter Two

Soups

Fresh, vibrant, healthy and generally low in carbohydrates and fat, soup is the perfect fuel for those watching their weight, without wanting to miss out on vital nutrients. As the following recipes demonstrate, soups are incredibly versatile. There are thick, hearty soups, which can be a meal in themselves, as well as lighter broths, which make excellent appetizers or even snacks, taking the edge off hunger pangs. There are also chilled soups for the hotter summer months. Two recipes for homemade stock are included in this chapter: one chicken (see page 22) and one vegetable (see page 23). These can be used as the base for all the soup recipes. Homemade stocks contain minimal amounts of carbohydrate, while store-bought alternatives vary in their content and can even be alarmingly high because some contain carbohydrate-based fillers and additives. If buying ready-made stocks do check the label first. Vegetable bouillon powders are the best alternative to homemade. Most of the soups in this chapter freeze well, so it makes sense to make double and freeze the surplus, but avoid freezing those that contain fish or shellfish.

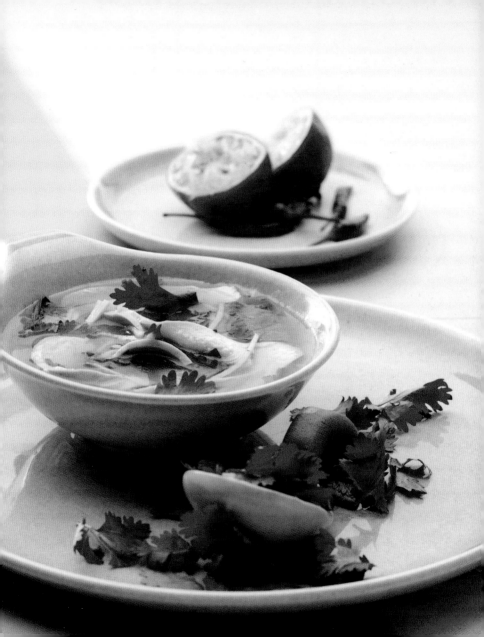

009

THAI CHICKEN BROTH SERVES 2

850ml/1½ pints/3½ cups chicken stock
(see recipe below)

1 stick lemongrass, peeled, halved
lengthways and crushed with a knife

4 slices fresh ginger, plus 2 slices, peeled
and cut into matchsticks

4 kaffir lime leaves

2 tsp Thai fish sauce

2 chicken breasts, about 140g/5oz each

2 cloves garlic, thinly sliced

35g/1¼oz/⅔ cup fresh spinach leaves

2 tbsp rice vinegar

1 tbsp lime juice

1 bird's eye chilli, seeded and finely
chopped

1 tbsp chopped fresh coriander/cilantro

1   Put the stock, lemongrass, 4 ginger slices, lime leaves and fish sauce into a
    saucepan. Add the chicken breasts and bring to the boil. Reduce the heat and
    simmer, half-covered, for 20 minutes. Remove the chicken, set aside, and strain the
    stock, discarding the solids.
2   Return the stock to the pan and add the ginger matchsticks, garlic, spinach, rice
    vinegar, lime juice and chilli, then simmer for 2–3 minutes.
3   Slice the chicken into strips and divide between 2 bowls. Pour over the stock.
    Season with salt, if necessary, and garnish with fresh coriander/cilantro.

7G CARBOHYDRATE PER SERVING

CHICKEN STOCK MAKES ABOUT 850ML/1½ PINTS/3½ CUPS

1 chicken carcass

1 onion, roughly chopped

1 carrot, roughly chopped

1 stick celery, roughly chopped

1 bay leaf

6 black peppercorns

handful of fresh parsley

1.5 litres/2¾ pints/6½ cups water

Place all the ingredients in a deep, narrow
saucepan, making sure they are covered by the
water, and bring to the boil. Reduce the heat and
simmer, uncovered, for 1½ hours, skimming off any
fat that rises to the surface. Replenish with more
cold water if the ingredients become uncovered.
Strain the stock and discard the solids. Leave to cool,
pour the stock into a container and store in the
refrigerator for up to 3 days or freeze until required.

Thai Chicken Broth pictured on page 21

010

SPINACH & PEA SOUP SERVES 2

1 tbsp olive oil
1 onion, finely chopped
1 carrot, finely chopped
850ml/1½ pints/3½ cups vegetable
stock (see recipe below)
150g/5½oz/1 cup frozen petit pois

175g/6oz/2¾ cups fresh spinach, tough
stalks removed
1 tbsp chopped fresh mint
salt and freshly ground black pepper
2 tbsp reduced-fat crème fraiche,
to serve

1   Heat the oil in a saucepan and fry the onion for 7 minutes, stirring frequently,
    until softened. Add the carrot and cook for a further 3 minutes.
2   Pour in the stock and bring to the boil. Reduce the heat and simmer for
    10 minutes.
3   Add the petit pois, spinach and mint and cook for 3 minutes until the vegetables
    are tender. Transfer to a blender and process until smooth. Season and serve with
    a spoonful of crème fraiche.

13G CARBOHYDRATE PER SERVING

VEGETABLE STOCK MAKES ABOUT 850ML/1½ PINTS/3½ CUPS

2 onions, cut into 1cm/½in dice
2 carrots, cut into 1cm/½in dice
2 sticks celery, cut into 1cm/½in dice
1 leek, cut into 1cm/½in dice
1 bay leaf
2 sprigs fresh thyme
handful of fresh parsley
1.5 litres/2¾ pints/6½ cups water

Place all the ingredients in a deep, narrow
saucepan, making sure all the ingredients
are covered by the water. Bring the water to
the boil, then reduce the heat and simmer for
40 minutes, skimming off any scum that rises
to the surface. Strain the stock and discard
the solids. Leave to cool, pour the stock into a
container and store in the refrigerator for
up to 3 days or freeze until required.

011

PISTOU SERVES 2

1 tbsp olive oil
1 leek, sliced
1 small carrot, finely chopped
1 stick celery, finely chopped
3 green beans, thinly sliced
700ml/1¼ pints/3 cups vegetable stock (see page 23)
150ml/5fl oz/⅔ cup passata
1 bay leaf

30g/1oz/½ cup whole-wheat conchigliette (small shells) pasta
30g/1oz/½ cup canned cannellini beans, rinsed
sprig of fresh rosemary
salt and freshly ground black pepper
a few shavings of Parmesan, to serve
1 tbsp pesto, to serve

1   Heat the oil in a large saucepan and add the leek. Cook over a medium heat for 5 minutes, stirring occasionally, until tender. Add the carrot, celery and green beans and cook for a further 5 minutes.

2   Pour in the stock and passata and add the bay leaf, stir well. Bring to the boil, then reduce the heat and simmer, half-covered, for 15 minutes. Remove the bay leaf and using a hand-blender or food processor, semi-purée the vegetables.

3   Return the bay leaf to the soup, add the pasta, cannellini beans, and rosemary and bring to the boil. Reduce the heat slightly and cook for 10 minutes or until the pasta is tender. You may need to add some extra stock or water if the soup seems too thick. Remove the bay leaf and rosemary and season to taste.

4   Divide between 2 bowls. Serve with the Parmesan shavings and a spoonful of pesto.

19G CARBOHYDRATE PER SERVING

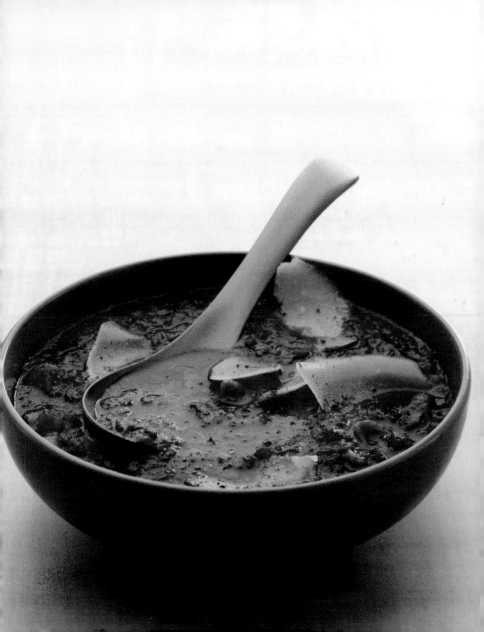

012

ROASTED TOMATO & ROSEMARY SOUP SERVES 2

6 vine-ripened plum tomatoes

2 tbsp olive oil

1 leek, sliced

1 clove garlic, chopped

2 sprigs fresh rosemary

1 bay leaf

100ml/3½fl oz/½ cup passata

600ml/1 pint/2½ cups vegetable stock
  (see page 23)

salt and freshly ground black pepper

1   Preheat the oven to 180°C/350°F/Gas 4. Put the tomatoes in a roasting pan with
    half of the oil and roast for 20 minutes until tender. Leave until cool enough to
    handle, then peel away the skin and deseed. Chop the flesh.

2   Heat the remaining oil in a heavy saucepan and fry the leek for 4 minutes until
    softened. Add the garlic, rosemary and bay leaf and cook for a further 1 minute.

3   Pour in the passata and stock, then bring to the boil. Reduce the heat and
    simmer for 15 minutes until thickened. Add the chopped tomatoes and cook
    for a further 5 minutes.

4   Remove the rosemary and bay leaf and transfer the soup to a blender. Process
    until smooth and season well.

7G CARBOHYDRATE PER SERVING

013

VIETNAMESE BEEF BROTH SERVES 2

850ml/1¹/₂ pints/3¹/₂ cups vegetable
  stock (see page 23) or beef stock
1 tbsp fish sauce
2 star anise
2 bird's eye chillies, seeded and halved
2.5cm/1in piece fresh ginger, peeled
  and sliced
1 stick lemongrass, peeled and crushed
2 cloves garlic, sliced

2 kaffir lime leaves
250g/9oz lean fillet beef, thinly sliced
1 large head pak choi/bok choy
100g/3¹/₂oz/1¹/₃ cups bean sprouts
juice of 1 lime
1 tsp soy sauce
2 spring onions/scallions, finely sliced
15g/¹/₂oz/¹/₂ cup chopped fresh
  coriander/cilantro

1   Put the stock, fish sauce, star anise, chillies, ginger, lemongrass, garlic and lime
    leaves in a saucepan. Bring to the boil, then reduce the heat and simmer for
    15 minutes. Strain, discard the solids, and return the flavoured stock to the pan.
2   Add the beef and cook for 4 minutes, then add the pak choi/bok choy and
    bean sprouts and cook for a further 2 minutes. Stir in the lime juice and soy sauce,
    spring onions/scallions and coriander/cilantro.

7G CARBOHYDRATE PER SERVING

014

GAZPACHO WITH AVOCADO SALSA SERVES 2

1 handful of cashew nuts

450g/1lb vine-ripened tomatoes, peeled, seeded and chopped

1 small cucumber, peeled, seeded and chopped

1 small red pepper, seeded and chopped

1 green chilli, seeded and sliced

1 clove garlic, crushed

1 tbsp extra-virgin olive oil

juice of 1 lime

few drops Tabasco sauce

salt and freshly ground black pepper

4 ice cubes, to serve

chopped fresh basil, to serve

AVOCADO SALSA:

1 ripe avocado, pitted, peeled and diced

1 tsp lemon juice

2.5cm/1in piece cucumber, diced

½ red chilli, finely chopped

1   Soak the cashew nuts in a little water for 1 hour. Place the cashews with the tomatoes, cucumber, red pepper, chilli, garlic, oil, lime juice and Tabasco in a food processor or blender. Add 250ml/9fl oz/1 cup of water and blend until combined but still chunky. Season to taste and chill for 2–3 hours.

2   Just before serving make the avocado salsa. Toss the avocado in the lemon juice to prevent it browning. Combine with the cucumber and chilli.

3   Ladle the soup into bowls, add the ice cubes, and top with a spoonful of salsa. Garnish with the basil just before serving.

10G CARBOHYDRATE PER SERVING

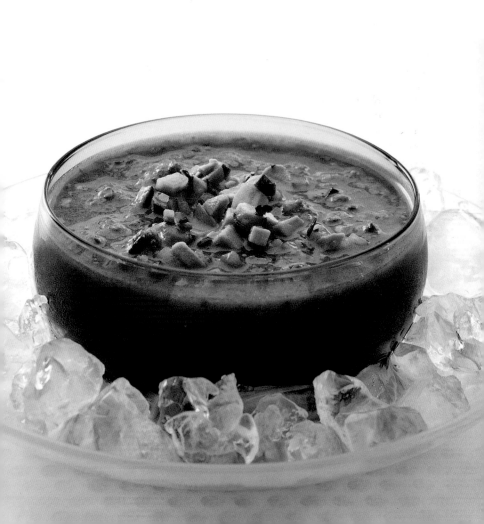

015

SPICY FISH & CHICKPEA SOUP

SERVES 2

2 tbsp sunflower oil

2 onions, finely sliced

3 cardamom pods, seeds removed

1 tsp cumin seeds

1 tsp ground coriander

1cm/½in piece fresh ginger, peeled and grated

1 red chilli, seeded and finely sliced

2 large cloves garlic, crushed

1 bay leaf

225g/8oz/1⅓ cups peeled and cubed butternut squash

600ml/1 pint/2½ cups vegetable stock (see page 23)

salt and freshly ground black pepper

squeeze of lemon juice

70g/2½oz/⅓ cup canned chickpeas/garbanzo beans, rinsed

2 thick cod fillets, skinned, about 200g/7oz each

2 tbsp natural bio yogurt, to serve

1 tbsp chopped fresh coriander/cilantro, to serve

1   Heat half the oil in a large saucepan and fry one of the onions for 7 minutes until softened. Add the seeds, spices, garlic and bay leaf and cook for another minute.

2   Add the squash and stock to the pan. Bring to the boil, then reduce the heat and simmer, half-covered, for 10–12 minutes until the squash is tender. Remove the bay leaf and blend until puréed. Season to taste, add a squeeze of lemon juice and the chickpeas/garbanzo beans and cook for a further 5 minutes, half-covered.

3   Meanwhile, preheat the grill/broiler to its highest setting. Line a grill/broiler pan with foil, then lightly oil. Season the fish, then grill/broil for about 4–5 minutes each side.

4   Heat the remaining oil in a frying pan and fry the second onion until crisp.

5   Ladle the soup into 2 shallow bowls and top with the fish fillets. Place a spoonful of yogurt on top of the fish, then sprinkle with the crisp onion and coriander/cilantro.

22G CARBOHYDRATE PER SERVING

016

SMOKED HADDOCK CHOWDER

SERVES 2

300g/10½oz undyed smoked haddock
    fillets
55g/2oz/¼ cup split red lentils, rinsed
1 bay leaf
1 leek, sliced
1 carrot, sliced
1 stick celery, sliced

850ml/1½ pints/3½ cups vegetable
    stock (see page 23)
55g/2oz/⅓ cup drained and rinsed
    canned no-sugar-or-salt sweetcorn/
    corn kernels
3 tbsp reduced-fat crème fraîche
salt and freshly ground black pepper
1 tbsp snipped fresh chives, to serve

1   Place the haddock in a sauté pan and cover with water. Poach for 8 minutes
    or until cooked. Remove the fish from the poaching liquid using a fish slice and
    leave to cool. Remove the skin and any bones and flake the flesh into large
    pieces; set aside.
2   Place the lentils, bay leaf, leek, carrot, celery and stock in a large saucepan. Bring
    to the boil, skim off any scum that rises to the surface and reduce the heat. Simmer
    for 25 minutes, half-covered, until the lentils and vegetables are tender, adding
    the corn 5 minutes before the end of the cooking time.
3   Remove the bay leaf and transfer the soup to a blender. Process until half-puréed
    but still chunky. Return the soup to the pan and stir in the crème fraîche. Gently stir
    in the haddock, making sure you don't break up the chunks and season to taste.
    Heat gently, then serve sprinkled with the chives.

15G CARBOHYDRATE PER SERVING

Chapter Three

Salads, Light Meals & Snacks

This chapter features a range of recipes that suit a number of different eating occasions, whether you are looking for a quick, healthy snack, a light lunch or a simple supper dish. It can be tricky to find snacks that are not carbohydrate-based (healthy or not). It's all too easy to grab a slice of white bread, a biscuit/cookie or handful of crisps/potato chips when feeling hungry and time is short. But when it comes to snacking, look at foods that perhaps you wouldn't necessarily regard as a typical snack, such as a hard-boiled egg, a slice of ham, canned fish, a handful of nuts or seeds, vegetable crudités or an open sandwich piled high with filling, rather than the usual two-slice version with a small amount of filling. Many of the following light meals can be made in advance or can form the base of a larger main meal when paired with a salad or moderate amount of noodles or brown rice. Salads don't have to be sidelined as an accompaniment – many of the recipes here contain a protein element, such as lean meat, poultry, seafood, nuts, seeds, cheese or eggs, helping satiate the appetite. All of the salad recipes come with their own dressing. It's well worth taking the time to make your own dressings; not only to suit your own taste but in order to control what goes into them.

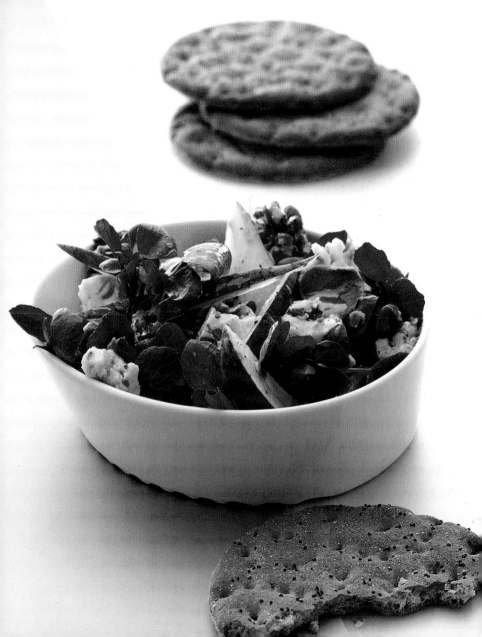

017

WATERCRESS, WALNUT & ROQUEFORT SALAD SERVES 2

1 small red William pear, cored
   and sliced
1 tsp lemon juice
55g/2oz/½ cup walnut halves
140g/5oz/1⅔ bunches watercress, tough
   stalks removed
115g/4oz/1 cup cubed Roquefort cheese

DRESSING:
2 tbsp extra-virgin olive oil
1 tbsp lemon juice
½ tsp Dijon mustard
salt and freshly ground black pepper

1   Toss the pear slices in the lemon juice to prevent them browning. Toast the
    walnuts in a dry frying pan for 2 minutes.
2   To make the dressing, whisk together the oil, lemon juice and mustard,
    then season.
3   Arrange the watercress in a bowl and top with the pear slices, Roquefort and
    walnuts. Pour over the dressing, toss well and serve.

11G CARBOHYDRATE PER SERVING

SALADS, LIGHT MEALS & SNACKS

Recipe pictured on page 33

018

BEAN & ROASTED RED PEPPER SALAD SERVES 2

1 red pepper, seeded and
  quartered
2½ tbsp extra-virgin olive oil
1 clove garlic, crushed
3 tbsp chopped fresh oregano

2 tsp balsamic vinegar
150g/5½oz/1 cup drained and rinsed
  canned butter/lima beans
salt and freshly ground black pepper

1 Preheat the oven to 200°C/400°F/Gas 6. Place the pepper on a baking sheet,
   brush with some of the oil and roast for 20–25 minutes until tender and blackened
   around the edges. Set aside until cool enough to handle.
2 Peel the red pepper then cut into small bite-size pieces.
3 Gently heat the remaining oil in a saucepan and cook the garlic for 1 minute.
   Remove from the heat and stir in the oregano, vinegar and the red pepper.
4 Put the beans in a serving bowl and pour the red pepper mixture over. Season
   well and stir until the beans are coated in the mixture.

13G CARBOHYDRATE PER SERVING

019

MELON & FETA SALAD SERVES 2

2 wedges melon, preferably Charentais
 or Cantaloupe, peeled and cut into
 cubes
85g/3oz/²⁄₃ cup cubed feta cheese
mint leaves, to garnish

DRESSING:
1 tbsp lemon juice
1½ tbsp extra-virgin olive oil
freshly ground black pepper

1   Arrange the melon and feta on a platter. Whisk together the lemon juice and oil
    and pour it over the melon and feta. Season with pepper and garnish with mint.

8G CARBOHYDRATE PER SERVING

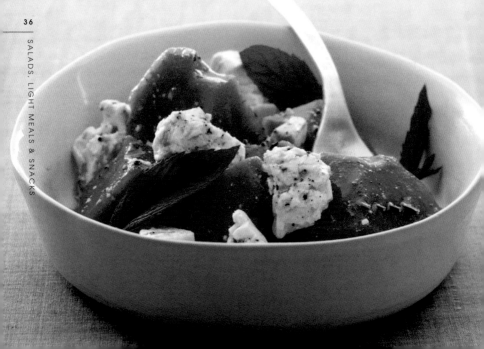

020

GRILLED AUBERGINE SALAD SERVES 2

1 aubergine/eggplant, sliced
2 tbsp extra-virgin olive oil

DRESSING:

2 tbsp extra-virgin olive oil
1 tbsp lemon juice
2 tbsp chopped fresh mint
salt and freshly ground black pepper

1   Steam the aubergine/eggplant for 6 minutes, then drain well and pat dry with
    paper towels.
2   Preheat the grill/broiler to medium and line the grill/broiler pan with foil. Place
    the aubergine/eggplant in the grill/broiler pan and brush the top with a little oil.
    Grill/broil for 2–3 minutes, then turn over, brush with more oil and return to the
    grill/broiler for 2–3 minutes until the slices are tender and golden.
3   Meanwhile, mix together the ingredients for the dressing; season.
4   Put the aubergine/eggplant in a shallow dish, pour the dressing over and
    serve warm.

3G CARBOHYDRATE PER SERVING

SALADS, LIGHT MEALS & SNACKS

021

AVOCADO, RED ONION & SPINACH SALAD SERVES 2

2 tsp extra-virgin olive oil

1 red onion, cut into wedges

100g/3½oz/1¾ cups baby spinach
leaves

1 avocado, peeled, pitted and sliced

a little lemon juice

DRESSING:

2 tbsp extra-virgin olive oil, plus extra
for greasing

1–2 tsp balsamic vinegar, to taste

salt and freshly ground black pepper

1   Preheat the oven to 200°C/400°F/Gas 6. Pour the olive oil into a baking dish and add the onion wedges. Bake for 25 minutes, turning occasionally, until the onion is tender. Leave to cool.

2   To make the dressing, whisk together the oil and vinegar, then season.

3   Arrange the spinach in a serving bowl. Toss the avocado in lemon juice and add to the bowl with the onion. Pour over the dressing and toss gently.

6G CARBOHYDRATE PER SERVING

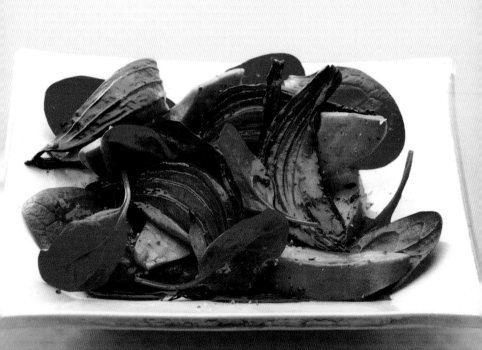

022

GREEK SALAD SERVES 2

85g/3oz/⅔ cup cubed feta cheese
3 vine-ripened tomatoes, seeded and
  cut into chunks
10cm/4in piece cucumber, cut into
  chunks
55g/2oz/⅓ cup black olives

1 tsp dried oregano
freshly ground black pepper

DRESSING:
2 tbsp extra-virgin olive oil
1 tbsp lemon juice

1 Place the feta, tomatoes, cucumber and black olives in a serving bowl.
2 Whisk together the olive oil and lemon juice and pour the dressing over the salad.
    Toss with your hands to coat the salad in the dressing.
3 Sprinkle with the oregano and season with black pepper before serving.

9G CARBOHYDRATE PER SERVING

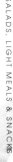

023

JAPANESE-STYLE SMOKED TOFU SALAD SERVES 2

55g/2oz buckwheat noodles
200g/7oz block smoked tofu
85g/3oz/1 cup finely shredded white
  cabbage
1 small carrot, finely shredded
2 spring onions/scallions, sliced
1 green chilli, seeded and finely sliced
  into rounds
1 tbsp sesame seeds, toasted
salt and freshly ground black pepper

DRESSING:
1 tsp grated fresh ginger
1 clove garlic, crushed
2 tbsp silken tofu
2 tsp soy sauce
1 tbsp sesame oil
2 tbsp hot water

1   Cook the noodles in plenty of boiling salted water following the package
    instructions. Drain and refresh under cold running water.
2   Blend all the ingredients for the dressing until smooth and creamy; season.
3   Drain the tofu and steam for 5 minutes, then cut into long, thin slices.
4   Mix together the cabbage, carrot, onions and chilli. To serve, arrange
    the noodles on two plates, then top with the vegatables and slices of tofu.
    Spoon over the dressing and sprinkle with sesame seeds.

24.5G CARBOHYDRATE PER SERVING

024

COURGETTE & HALLOUMI
SALAD SERVES 2

5 small courgettes/zucchini, sliced
   lengthways
6 slices halloumi cheese

DRESSING:
2 tbsp extra-virgin olive oil
1 tbsp lemon juice
1 tbsp chopped fresh flat-leaf parsley
1 tbsp capers, rinsed

1   Steam the courgettes/zucchini for 1–2 minutes until just tender. Refresh under cold
    running water and drain well.

2   Blend together the ingredients for the dressing. Arrange the courgettes/zucchini in
    a shallow dish and pour the dressing over.

3   Heat a griddle pan until hot. Place the halloumi in the pan and cook for about
    2 minutes each side until golden. Arrange on top of the courgettes/zucchini.

6G CARBOHYDRATE PER SERVING

025

QUINOA TABBOULEH SERVES 2

55g/2oz/¼ cup quinoa

3 vine-ripened small tomatoes, seeded
and chopped

5cm/2in piece cucumber, diced

2 spring onions/scallions, finely
chopped

2 tbsp lemon juice

1 tbsp extra-virgin olive oil

2 tbsp chopped fresh mint

2 tbsp chopped fresh coriander/cilantro

2 tbsp chopped fresh parsley

salt and freshly ground black pepper

1   Cover the quinoa with 200ml/7fl oz/1 cup water and bring to the boil. Reduce the
    heat, cover, and simmer over a low heat for about 10–15 minutes or until tender.
    Drain if necessary.

2   Leave the quinoa to cool slightly before combining with the rest of the ingredients.
    Season well before serving at room temperature.

24G CARBOHYDRATE PER SERVING

026

BROAD BEAN, PRAWN & AVOCADO SALAD SERVES 2

100g/3½oz/⅔ cup shelled broad/fava
   beans
1 avocado, peeled, pitted and sliced
1 tsp lemon juice
2 handfuls mixed salad leaves
175g/6oz/1 cup shelled cooked king
   prawns/jumbo shrimp
1 tbsp chopped chives

DRESSING:
1 tbsp extra-virgin olive oil
2 tsp lemon juice
1 tbsp creamed horseradish sauce
1 tbsp reduced-fat crème fraîche
salt and freshly ground black pepper

1   Steam the broad/fava beans for 3–4 minutes until tender. Leave to cool slightly,
    then remove the tough outer skin from each bean. Meanwhile, toss the avocado
    in the lemon juice to prevent it from browning.
2   To make the dressing, whisk together the oil, lemon juice, creamed horseradish
    and crème fraîche. Season well.
3   Arrange the salad leaves in 2 shallow bowls and add the avocado, broad/fava
    beans and prawns/shrimp. Pour over the dressing, toss gently, and sprinkle with
    chives before serving.

7G CARBOHYDRATE PER SERVING

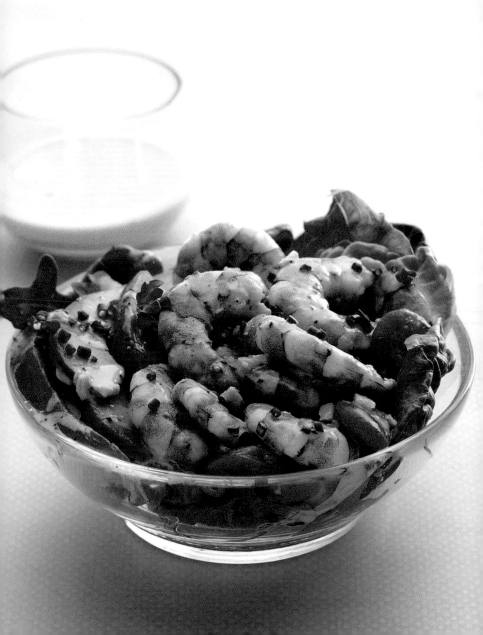

027

CRAB SALAD WITH HERB MAYO

SERVES 2

8 spears asparagus, trimmed
2 handfuls mixed salad leaves
2 dressed crabs

HERB MAYO:
1 tbsp extra-virgin olive oil
2 tbsp reduced-fat mayonnaise
1 tbsp fresh basil
1 tbsp fresh oregano
1 tbsp fresh chives
salt and freshly ground black pepper

1　Put the ingredients for the herb mayo in a blender and process until smooth and creamy. Season.
2　Steam the asparagus for about 5 minutes or until tender.
3　Divide the salad leaves between two plates. Scoop out the crabmeat and place on top of the leaves. Top with the asparagus. Serve with the herb mayonnaise.

2G CARBOHYDRATE PER SERVING

028

SMOKED TROUT SALAD WITH DILL DRESSING SERVES 2

70g/2½oz/1½ cups spinach, rocket/
   arugula and watercress salad
1 shallot, diced
5cm/2in piece cucumber, coarsely
   grated
2 cooked beetroot/beets in natural
   juice, drained and diced
½ avocado, pitted, peeled and sliced
2 smoked trout fillets

DRESSING:
1 tbsp extra-virgin olive oil
1 tbsp reduced-fat mayonnaise
1½ tbsp dill sauce
1 tbsp warm water
freshly ground black pepper

1   Mix together all the ingredients for the dressing, then season with pepper.
2   Place the salad leaves on 2 serving plates, then arrange the shallot, cucumber,
   beetroot/beets and avocado on top.
3   Place a trout fillet on top of each salad and drizzle over the dressing.

8G CARBOHYDRATE PER SERVING

029

FRESH TUNA NIÇOISE SERVES 2

1 tbsp extra-virgin olive oil

1 tbsp lemon juice

2 tuna steaks, 140g/5oz each

85g/3oz fine green beans, cooked

2 handfuls mixed salad leaves

6 cherry tomatoes, halved

1/2 small red onion, sliced

1 hard-boiled egg, chopped

handful of pitted black olives

salt and freshly ground black pepper

DRESSING:

1 tbsp extra-virgin olive oil

1/2 tsp white wine vinegar

1 small clove garlic, crushed

3 tsp reduced-fat mayonnaise

1   Mix together the oil and lemon juice and season well. Place the tuna in a shallow dish and pour over the marinade. Cover and chill for 30 minutes, turning occasionally.

2   Put the green beans, salad leaves, tomatoes, onion, egg and olives in a bowl.

3   Whisk together the ingredients for the dressing, then pour it over the salad and toss well using your hands.

4   Heat a griddle or frying pan until hot. Place the tuna steaks in the pan, brush with the marinade and cook for 5 minutes, turning once, until cooked on the outside and pink in the middle. Brush with the marinade when needed.

5   Arrange the salad on serving plates and top each one with a tuna steak.

7G CARBOHYDRATE PER SERVING

Recipe pictured on page 5

030

SQUID SALAD WITH HERB DRESSING SERVES 2

extra-virgin olive oil, for brushing

250g/9oz fresh prepared squid, cleaned and each one cut into 3

85g/3oz/1¾ cups rocket/arugula

3 tomatoes, seeded and chopped

DRESSING:

2 tbsp chopped fresh basil

1 tbsp chopped fresh oregano

1 tbsp chopped fresh chives

2 tbsp extra-virgin olive oil

2 tsp lemon juice

1 clove garlic, crushed

salt and freshly ground black pepper

1   Blend the ingredients for the dressing in a food processor or blender. Season to taste and set aside.

2   Brush a griddle pan with oil and cook the squid over a medium-high heat for 1½ minutes, turning halfway.

3   Put the rocket/arugula and tomatoes in a shallow dish. Add the squid and spoon over the dressing. Toss until the salad is coated in the dressing.

3G CARBOHYDRATE PER SERVING

031

CHICKEN SALAD WITH SPICY
AVOCADO DRESSING <small>SERVES 2</small>

2 skinless chicken breasts, 175g/6oz each

1 tbsp extra-virgin olive oil

1 small yellow pepper, seeded and
sliced

2 handfuls mixed rocket/arugula,
spinach and watercress leaves

12 cherry tomatoes, halved

2 spring onions/scallions, sliced
diagonally

salt and freshly ground black pepper

1 tbsp fresh coriander/cilantro leaves,
to garnish

DRESSING:

1 avocado, peeled, pitted and chopped

zest and juice of 1 lime

3 tbsp fromage frais

1 tbsp chopped coriander/cilantro

¼ tsp dried crushed chilli flakes

1   Put the chicken breasts between 2 sheets of cling film/plastic wrap and flatten
with the end of a rolling pin. Heat a griddle pan and brush with the oil. Season the
chicken and griddle for about 2–4 minutes each side, depending on the thickness
of the fillets, until cooked through. Remove from the pan and add the pepper and
cook for about 5 minutes until tender.

2   Blend together the ingredients for the dressing and season well.

3   Peel the pepper slices. Arrange the salad leaves on 2 plates, then add the
pepper, tomatoes and spring onions/scallions. Spoon over the dressing. Slice the
chicken and place on top of the salad, then sprinkle with coriander/cilantro.

10G CARBOHYDRATE PER SERVING

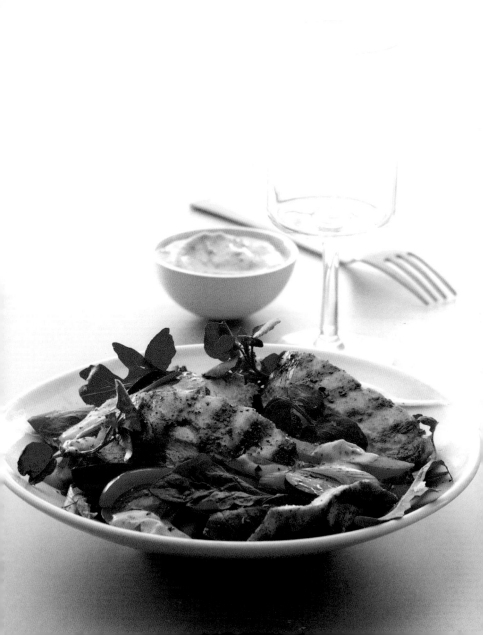

032

CHICKEN CAESAR SALAD SERVES 2

2 skinless chicken breasts, 125g/4½oz
  each, cut into strips

2 handfuls Cos lettuce, leaves torn into
  bite-size pieces

Parmesan shavings, to serve

DRESSING:

2 anchovy fillets

1½ tbsp extra-virgin olive oil, plus extra
  for brushing

1 tbsp reduced-fat mayonnaise

½ clove garlic

2 tsp lemon juice

¼ tsp Dijon mustard

¼ tsp Worcestershire sauce

2 tbsp finely grated Parmesan

salt and freshly ground black pepper

1   Blend the dressing ingredients until smooth and creamy. Season to taste.

2   Heat a griddle pan until hot. Brush the pan with oil and griddle the chicken for
    3–4 minutes each side until cooked through. Leave to cool slightly.

3   Put the lettuce leaves in a bowl and spoon over the dressing. Toss to coat the
    leaves. Put the chicken on top and sprinkle with Parmesan shavings.

2.5G CARBOHYDRATE PER SERVING

033

ITALIAN SALAD <small>SERVES 2</small>

2 portobello mushrooms, sliced
2 slices prosciutto
1 avocado
1 tsp lemon juice
70g/2½oz/1¼ cups baby spinach leaves
2 tbsp Parmesan shavings

DRESSING:
1 tbsp extra-virgin olive oil, plus extra
   for brushing
2 tbsp reduced-fat mayonnaise
2 anchovy fillets
1 tsp Dijon mustard
1 tsp lemon juice
salt and freshly ground black pepper

1   Preheat the grill/broiler to medium-high and line with foil. Brush the mushrooms
    with oil and grill/broil for about 5 minutes until starting to turn crisp. Grill/broil the
    prosciutto at the same time until crisp. Leave the mushrooms and prosciutto to
    cool slightly.
2   Peel, pit and slice the avocado and drizzle with the lemon juice to prevent it
    browning and put it in a bowl with the spinach. Slice and add the mushrooms.
3   Blend together the ingredients for the dressing and season to taste. Pour the
    dressing over the salad and toss to coat. Top with the prosciutto and Parmesan.

4.5G CARBOHYDRATE PER SERVING

034

PROSCIUTTO & MOZZARELLA
SALAD SERVES 2

2 yellow peppers, seeded and
  quartered
2 tbsp extra-virgin olive oil
150g/5½oz mozzarella, drained and torn
  into pieces

4 slices prosciutto, cut into 2.5cm/1in
  pieces
1 clove garlic, crushed
2 tsp balsamic vinegar
salt and freshly ground black pepper

1   Preheat the oven to 200°C/400°F/Gas 6. Brush the peppers with half of the oil.
    Place them on a baking sheet and roast for 25–30 minutes until tender and
    blackened around the edges. Leave to cool slightly, then peel off the skin.

2   Slice the peppers and place them in a bowl with the mozzarella and prosciutto.

3   Mix the garlic and vinegar with the remaining oil. Season to taste and pour it over
    the salad. Toss the salad in the dressing and serve.

7G CARBOHYDRATE PER SERVING

035

DUCK & ORANGE SALAD WITH WATERCRESS SERVES 2

150g/5½oz skinless duck breast
85g/3oz/1 bunch watercress
55g/2oz fennel, sliced
½ orange, peeled and sliced into
  rounds

DRESSING:
2 tbsp extra-virgin olive oil, plus extra
  for brushing
2 tbsp fresh orange juice
1 tbsp lemon juice
salt and freshly ground black pepper

1   Preheat the grill/broiler to high and line the grill/broiler pan with foil. Brush the
    duck with a little oil and season, then grill/broil for 4–5 minutes each side until
    cooked. Leave to rest for 3 minutes, then thinly slice.
2   Mix together the ingredients for the dressing, then season.
3   Arrange the watercress and sliced fennel on a serving plate, then top with the
    orange slices. Place the duck on top and then gently spoon the dressing over.

7.5G CARBOHYDRATE PER SERVING

SALADS, LIGHT MEALS & SNACKS

036

THAI-STYLE BEEF SALAD SERVES 2

300g/10½oz rump steak, cut into
  1cm/½in strips
1 tbsp olive oil
2 Little Gem lettuces, leaves separated
2 shallots, finely sliced
150g/5½oz vine-ripened tomatoes,
  quartered
1 bird's eye chilli, seeded and
  finely sliced
2 tbsp fresh coriander/cilantro leaves
1 tbsp torn fresh basil
salt and freshly ground black pepper

DRESSING:
juice of 1 lime
½ tsp honey
1 tbsp extra-virgin olive oil
1 clove garlic, crushed
1 tbsp Thai fish sauce
2 tsp soy sauce

SALADS, LIGHT MEALS & SNACKS

1 Put the beef in a bowl with the oil and season well. Heat a frying pan and fry the
   beef for 4–5 minutes. Leave to cool slightly.

2 Arrange the salad leaves in 2 shallow dishes and top with the beef. Scatter over
   the shallots, tomatoes and chilli.

3 To make the dressing, mix together the lime juice and honey until it has dissolved,
   then stir in the oil, garlic, fish sauce and soy sauce. Pour the dressing over the
   salad. Season and sprinkle with the fresh herbs.

8G CARBOHYDRATE PER SERVING

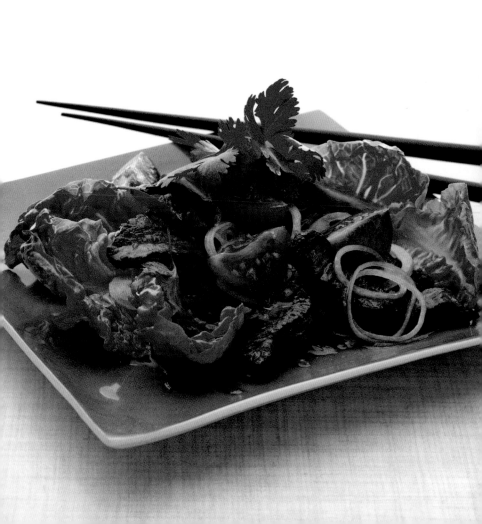

037

BROAD BEAN FALAFEL SERVES 4

140g/5oz/1 cup shelled broad/fava
  beans
125g/4½oz/⅔ cup canned chickpeas/
  garbanzo beans, rinsed
2 cloves garlic, crushed
2 spring onions/scallions, finely sliced
1 tsp ground cumin
½ tsp dried crushed chilli flakes

1 tsp ground coriander
1 tsp lemon juice
1 tbsp each fresh mint and parsley
½ egg, beaten
salt and freshly ground black pepper
soy flour, for dusting
sunflower oil, for frying

1   Steam the broad/fava beans for 2 minutes, then refresh under cold running water
    until cool.
2   Pop the beans out of their tough outer skins and put them in a food processor with
    the chickpeas/garbanzo beans, garlic, spring onions/scallions, spices, lemon juice,
    herbs and egg. Season well and blend until the mixture forms a coarse paste. Chill
    for 1 hour to allow the mixture to firm up.
3   Form the mixture into 12 walnut-size balls using floured hands, then roll in flour until
    lightly coated. Shake to remove any excess flour.
4   Heat 1 tablespoon of oil in a frying pan and cook the falafel in batches (adding
    more oil if necessary) for 6 minutes, turning occasionally, until golden. Drain on
    paper towels.

9G CARBOHYDRATE PER SERVING

038

SPICY TOFU CAKES SERVES 3

250g/9oz block firm tofu, drained,
   patted dry and grated
1 tbsp curry paste of your choice
1 large clove garlic, crushed
1 tbsp grated fresh ginger
½ tsp dried crushed chilli flakes

2 tbsp chopped fresh coriander/cilantro
2 spring onions/scallions, finely
   chopped
1½ tbsp soy flour, plus extra for shaping
salt
1 tbsp sunflower oil, for frying

1   Mix the tofu with the curry paste, garlic, ginger, chilli, coriander/cilantro and spring
    onions/scallions in a bowl. Stir in the flour and a pinch of salt to make a coarse,
    sticky paste. Refrigerate, covered, for 1 hour to allow the mixture to firm up slightly.
2   Take large walnut-size balls of the mixture and, using floured hands, flatten into
    rounds until you have 6 patties.
3   Heat the oil in a frying pan and cook the tofu cakes for 4–6 minutes, turning once,
    until golden. Drain on paper towels and serve warm.

3G CARBOHYDRATE PER SERVING

039

ORIENTAL OMELETTE PARCEL

SERVES 2

115g/4oz/1 cup small broccoli florets
1cm/$\frac{1}{2}$in piece fresh ginger, peeled
and finely grated
1 large clove garlic, crushed
2 red chillies, seeded and thinly sliced
2 tbsp sunflower oil
4 spring onions/scallions, sliced on
the diagonal

115g/4oz/1$\frac{3}{4}$ cup bean sprouts
1 large head pak choi/bok choy,
shredded
2 tbsp chopped fresh coriander/cilantro
3 tbsp black bean sauce
3 eggs, beaten
salt and freshly ground black pepper

1   Blanch the broccoli in boiling water for 2 minutes, drain, then refresh under cold
running water.
2   Meanwhile, stir-fry the ginger, garlic and half of the chilli in 1 tablespoon of the oil
for 1 minute. Add the spring onions/scallions, broccoli, bean sprouts and pak choi/
bok choy and stir-fry for 2 minutes, tossing the vegetables continuously. Add the
black bean sauce and half of the coriander/cilantro and heat through. Set aside
and keep warm.
3   Heat a little of the remaining oil in a frying pan and add a third of the beaten egg.
Swirl the egg until it covers the base of the pan. Cook the eggs until set, then turn
out onto a plate and keep warm while you make two further omelettes, adding
more oil, when necessary.
4   To serve, spoon a third of the vegetable stir-fry down the middle of each omelette
and roll up loosely. Cut in half crossways on the diagonal so the filling is visible.
Garnish with coriander/cilantro leaves and a few slices of chilli.

8G CARBOHYDRATE PER SERVING

Recipe pictured on page 2

040

TUNA & LEEK TORTILLA SERVES 4

1 tbsp extra-virgin olive oil
1 large leek, finely sliced
200g/7oz canned tuna in spring water,
  drained

6 eggs, beaten
salt and freshly ground black pepper

1   Heat the oil in a medium-size, ovenproof frying pan, then fry the leek for
    5 minutes until softened. Stir in the tuna, retaining some chunks and making
    sure that the leek and tuna are evenly spread over the base of the pan.
2   Preheat the grill/broiler to medium. Season the beaten eggs and pour them
    carefully over the tuna and leek mixture. Cook over a medium heat for 5 minutes
    or until the eggs are just set and the base of the tortilla is golden.
3   Place the pan under the grill/broiler and cook the top of the tortilla for 3 minutes
    or until set and lightly golden. Serve cut into wedges.

1G CARBOHYDRATE PER SERVING

SALADS, LIGHT MEALS & SNACKS

041

GRAVADLAX OPEN SANDWICH

SERVES 2

2 slices rye bread

2 large lettuce leaves

4 wafer-thin slices cucumber

2 slices gravadlax

1 tbsp dill sauce

1 tbsp reduced-fat mayonnaise

1 tsp lemon juice

1 hard-boiled egg, quartered

freshly ground black pepper

a little chopped fresh dill, to garnish

1   Place the rye bread on a serving plate. Arrange a lettuce leaf and two slices of cucumber on top of each slice. Arrange the gravadlax on top.

2   Mix together the dill sauce, mayonnaise and lemon juice and spoon over the gravadlax. Top with the egg, season with pepper, and garnish with the dill.

18G CARBOHYDRATE PER SERVING

SALADS, LIGHT MEALS & SNACKS

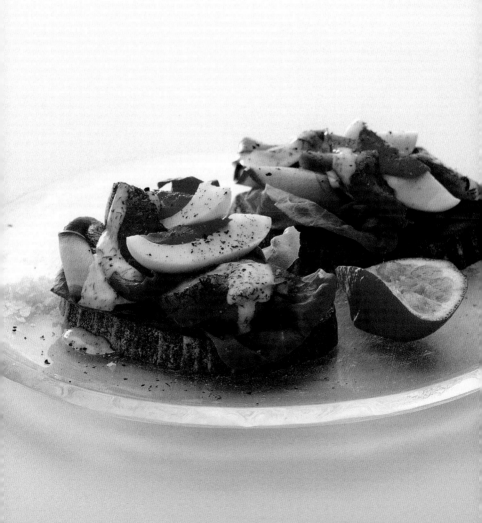

042

CRAB CAKES WITH CHILLI DIP

SERVES 2

140g/5oz/²⁄₃ cup fresh or canned white
  crab meat
115g/¼lb cod fillet, skinned and
  chopped
2 cloves garlic, chopped
¼ tsp dried crushed chilli flakes
1 stick lemongrass, peeled and finely
  chopped
1 tbsp finely grated fresh ginger

2 tbsp chopped fresh coriander/cilantro,
  plus extra to garnish
1 tbsp egg white
sunflower oil, for frying
salt and freshly ground black pepper

CHILLI DIP:
2 tbsp sweet chilli sauce
1 tbsp reduced-fat crème fraîche

SALADS, LIGHT MEALS & SNACKS

1 Blend the crab, cod, garlic, chilli, lemongrass, ginger, coriander/cilantro, egg
    white and seasoning in a food processor or blender until it forms a rough paste.
    Cover and chill for 30 minutes.

2 To make the dip, mix together the chilli sauce and crème fraîche.

3 Heat a little oil in a non-stick frying pan and place 3 heaped tablespoons of the
    crab paste in the pan, flattening the tops with a spatula. Fry for 3–4 minutes on
    each side until golden. Drain on paper towels and keep warm while you cook
    a further three cakes.

4 Serve three cakes per person with a spoonful of chilli dip. Garnish with
    coriander/cilantro.

14G CARBOHYDRATE PER SERVING

Recipe pictured on page 1

043

PAN-FRIED PRAWNS IN GARLIC

SERVES 2

8 large raw tiger prawns, peeled,
    deveined and tail left on
1 tbsp extra-virgin olive oil
1 tsp cayenne pepper

2 cloves garlic, chopped
1 tbsp chopped fresh parsley
salt and freshly ground black pepper

1   Put the prawns and half of the oil on a plate and sprinkle over the cayenne.
    Turn the prawns to coat them in the spiced oil.
2   Heat the remaining oil in a frying pan and add the prawns, spiced oil and garlic,
    then fry for about 3 minutes, turning once, until cooked. Season and sprinkle
    with parsley.

1G CARBOHYDRATE PER SERVING

044

CHICKEN SATAY MAKES 8 KEBABS

2 skinless chicken breasts, about
   140g/5oz each
1 tbsp extra-virgin olive oil
1 tbsp lemon juice
salt and freshly ground black pepper
fresh coriander/cilantro, leaves
   to garnish

SATAY SAUCE:
5 tbsp no-sugar smooth peanut butter
1 tbsp olive oil
1 tbsp hot water
1 tbsp soy sauce
1 tbsp fresh apple juice
2 tbsp reduced-fat coconut milk
1 red chilli, seeded and chopped

1   To make the satay sauce, mix together all the ingredients in a bowl.
2   Soak 8 wooden skewers in water for about 15 minutes to prevent them burning.
    Cut each breast into 4 strips lengthways and thread each one onto a skewer.
3   Combine the olive oil, lemon juice and seasoning in a small bowl, then brush the
    chicken with the marinade.
4   Heat a griddle pan or grill/broiler to medium-hot. Cook the chicken skewers
    for 3 minutes on each side until golden and cooked through, making sure there
    is no trace of pink inside. Serve the skewers with the satay sauce and garnished
    with coriander/cilantro.

6G CARBOHYDRATE PER KEBAB

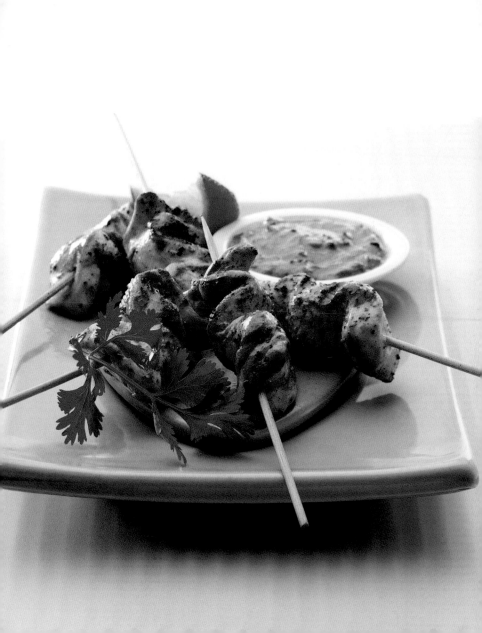

045

LAMB & TOMATO BRUSCHETTA

SERVES 1

1 lamb fillet, about 100g/3½oz

1 tbsp extra-virgin olive oil

2 tsp lemon juice

1 clove garlic, crushed

1 tsp dried oregano

1 small slice seeded wholemeal/
  whole-wheat bread, toasted

1 tsp Dijon mustard

1 tsp reduced-fat mayonnaise

handful of rocket/arugula leaves

1 vine-ripened tomato, sliced

salt and freshly ground black pepper

1   Flatten the lamb with the top of a rolling pin or meat mallet. Put the oil, lemon
    juice, garlic and oregano in a dish and add the lamb. Cover and marinate in the
    refrigerator for about 1 hour.

2   Preheat the grill/broiler to medium-high and line the grill/broiler pan with foil.
    Place the lamb in the pan and spoon over some of the marinade. Grill/broil for
    1–2 minutes each side.

3   Spread the toast with the mustard and mayonnaise. Place the rocket/arugula
    leaves on top, then the lamb and finally the tomato. Season well.

16.5G CARBOHYDRATE

046

CHILLI BEEF FAJITAS SERVES 2

1 tbsp extra-virgin olive oil
½ onion, thinly sliced
½ red pepper, seeded and sliced
¼ tsp dried crushed chilli flakes
½ tsp paprika
½ tsp ground cumin
125g/4½oz lean beef fillet, cut into
  thin strips

salt and freshly ground black pepper
4 Little Gem lettuce leaves
2 handfuls rocket/arugula leaves
juice of ½ lime
2 tsp sour cream, to serve
1 tbsp chopped fresh coriander/cilantro,
  to garnish

1   Heat the oil in a frying pan and fry the onion for 5 minutes, add the pepper and
    cook for another 3 minutes.
2   Add the spices and cook for 1 minute, before adding the beef. Season and cook,
    stirring frequently, for another 2 minutes.
3   Place the lettuce leaves on serving plates, top with the beef mixture and rocket/
    arugula and squeeze the lime juice over. Serve with a spoonful of sour cream and
    garnished with the coriander/cilantro.

3G CARBOHYDRATE PER SERVING

Chapter Four

Main Meals

Thailand, India, Spain, Italy, France and the Caribbean are just a few of the countries that have influenced the recipes in this chapter. This diversity of culinary ideas goes to show that low-carb cooking needn't be restrictive or dull. The chapter is broken down into sections on meat, poultry, seafood and vegetarian recipes. Many dishes come with a serving suggestion of a complex carbohydrate-based food, salad or vegetable depending on the level of carbohydrates in the main meal and the range of ingredients it includes. You'll also find suggestions for courgette/zucchini 'noodles', which can be made using a spiralizer or finely shredded with a knife, as well as cauliflower 'rice' (simply grated cauliflower florets) – and both can be served lightly steamed or raw, depending on your personal preference. The complex carbohydrate-based accompaniments include brown rice, whole-wheat pasta, couscous, buckwheat or soba noodles and have been chosen because they are unrefined, do not upset blood sugar levels and provide valuable fibre as well as vitamins and minerals. This does not mean you can over-indulge – 55g/2oz of each type is recommended. While you don't have to include this element when making the recipe, it gives an idea of how to prepare a balanced and nutritious meal.

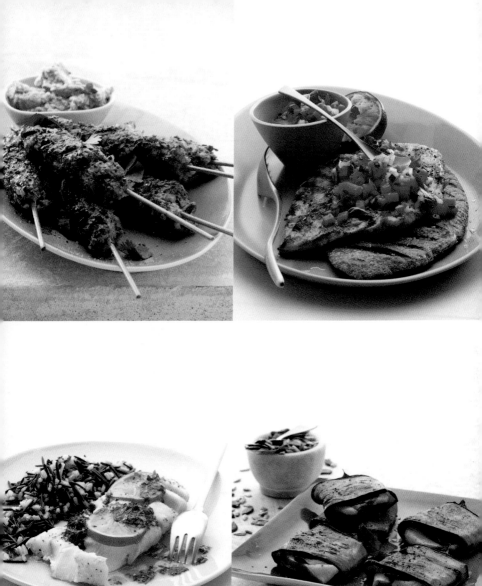

047

LAMB KOFTAS WITH CHICKPEA MASH SERVES 2 (MAKES 6 KOFTAS)

250g/9oz/packed 1 cup lean minced/ground lamb

1 onion, finely chopped

1 tbsp chopped fresh coriander/cilantro, plus extra to garnish

1 tbsp chopped fresh parsley

½ tsp ground coriander

¼ tsp chilli powder

salt and freshly ground black pepper

1 tbsp olive oil

1 recipe quantity Chickpea Mash (see page 127), to serve

1 Place the lamb, onion, fresh herbs, ground coriander, chilli and seasoning in a food processor. Blend until thoroughly combined.

2 Soak 6 wooden skewers in water for about 15 minutes to prevent them burning. Divide the lamb mixture into 6 portions and, using wet hands, shape each one into a sausage shape around a skewer. Cover and refrigerate the skewers for 30 minutes.

3 To cook, preheat a griddle pan and add the oil. Cook the skewers in two batches for 10 minutes, turning occasionally, or until browned on all sides and cooked through.

4 Sprinkle the koftas with chopped coriander/cilantro and serve with the Chickpea Mash.

2G CARBOHYDRATE PER SERVING • SERVE WITH A SIMPLE PEPPER SALAD

Recipe pictured on page 71 (top left)

048

ROAST MEDITERRANEAN LAMB

SERVES 4

1 clove garlic, sliced
2 tbsp chopped fresh oregano
2 tbsp chopped fresh rosemary
550g/1¼ lb boneless leg of lamb
4 bay leaves

2 tbsp olive oil
salt and freshly ground black pepper
8 small plum tomatoes
2 tbsp toasted pinenuts, to serve
   (optional)

1 Stuff the garlic, oregano and rosemary into the joint cavity and tuck the bay
   leaves under the string wrapped round the lamb. Rub half of the oil into the joint,
   season and leave, covered, in the refrigerator for 1–2 hours.

2 Preheat the oven to 190°C/375°F/Gas 5. Heat the remaining oil in a frying
   pan, add the lamb and brown the meat all over. Transfer the lamb to a roasting
   pan and cover with foil. Roast for 20 minutes, then remove the foil. Add 100ml/
   3½fl oz/½ cup of water to the pan to keep the lamb moist and cook for a further
   35 minutes, occasionally basting the meat in the cooking juices.

3 Arrange the tomatoes around the lamb 15 minutes before the end of the cooking
   time. Leave the meat to rest for 10 minutes, then carve into slices and serve with
   the tomatoes and pinenuts.

**7G CARBOHYDRATE PER SERVING • SERVE WITH ROASTED VEGETABLES AND STEAMED
GREEN BEANS**

049

HOMEMADE BEEF BURGER ON MUSHROOM MUFFIN SERVES 2

225g/8oz/1 cup lean minced/ground
   beef
1 large clove garlic, crushed
1 tsp dried oregano
2 large portobello mushrooms
2 tbsp olive oil
salt and freshly ground black pepper
2 thick slices beefsteak tomato, to serve
2 lettuce leaves, to serve

BLUE CHEESE DRESSING:
1 tbsp extra-virgin olive oil
1 tbsp reduced-fat mayonnaise
25g/1oz/¼ cup crumbled Roquefort
   cheese

1   Mix together the beef, garlic and oregano in a bowl. Season well and shape the
    mixture into 2 burgers. Cover with cling film/plastic wrap and chill for 30 minutes.
2   To make the blue cheese dressing, mix together the ingredients in a bowl.
3   Preheat the oven to 200°C/400°F/Gas 6. Put the mushrooms on a piece of foil
    large enough to make a parcel. Drizzle over half of the oil. Season and fold up the
    foil to make a parcel. Put the parcel on a baking sheet and cook for 20 minutes
    until softened.
4   Meanwhile, heat the remaining oil and fry the burgers over a medium heat
    for 4 minutes on each side.
5   To serve, place a mushroom on each plate, top with a slice of tomato, a lettuce
    leaf then the burger. Add a drizzle of blue cheese dressing before serving.

2G CARBOHYDRATE PER SERVING • SERVE WITH COLESLAW AND A GREEN SALAD

050

SLOW-COOKED INDONESIAN BEEF SERVES 2

1 tbsp groundnut oil
½ onion, finely chopped
300g/10½oz chuck steak, cut into
  4cm/1½in cubes
3 cloves garlic, chopped
1cm/½in fresh ginger, peeled and
  finely chopped
2 sticks lemongrass, peeled and
  crushed using the back of a knife
2 small red chillies, seeded and finely
  chopped

2 cardamom pods, split
2 tsp ground turmeric
½ tsp ground coriander
½ tsp chilli powder
½ tsp ground cumin
200ml/7fl oz/1 cup reduced-fat
  coconut milk
1 tbsp ground almonds
salt and freshly ground black pepper
2 tbsp desiccated coconut, toasted,
  to garnish

1 Heat the oil in a saucepan and fry the onion for 8 minutes, stirring occasionally, until softened. Add the meat and cook for 2–3 minutes each side until browned and sealed.
2 Add the garlic, ginger, lemongrass, chillies and all the spices and cook, stirring, for 1 minute.
3 Pour in the coconut milk and 125ml/4fl oz/½ cup water. Bring to the boil, then reduce the heat, cover, and simmer over a low heat for 2 hours. Add a little extra water if the curry seems too dry.
4 Uncover, add the almonds and cook for 5–10 minutes. Season to taste and serve sprinkled with the toasted coconut.

9.5G CARBOHYDRATE PER SERVING • SERVE WITH A SMALL BOWL OF BROWN
BASMATI RICE AND STEAMED PAK CHOI/BOK CHOY

051

AUTUMN BEEF STEW SERVES 4

2 tbsp soy flour
salt and freshly ground black pepper
800g/1¾lb casserole beef, cubed
3 tbsp olive oil
12 shallots, peeled and halved, or
quartered if large
1 carrot, cut into batons

85g/3oz/1 cup brown cap mushrooms,
halved
2 bay leaves
1 tbsp chopped fresh rosemary
450ml/16fl oz/2 cups red wine
200ml/7fl oz/1 cup beef stock
1 tbsp soy sauce

1 Preheat the oven to 170°C/325°F/Gas 3. Put the flour in a clean plastic food bag
   and season generously. Toss the beef in the flour until coated. Heat 1 tablespoon
   of the oil in a large casserole dish. Cook the beef in batches of about a third for
   5–6 minutes, turning occasionally, until browned all over. Add another tablespoon
   of oil as necessary. Set aside.

2 Add the remaining oil to the pan with the shallots, carrot, mushrooms and herbs
   and cook for 3 minutes, stirring occasionally.

3 Pour in the wine and bring to the boil. Cook over a high heat until the alcohol has
   evaporated and the liquid reduced. Add the stock and soy sauce then cook for
   another 3 minutes.

4 Stir in the beef, cover with a lid, and transfer to the oven. Cook for 2 hours until
   the stock has formed a thick, rich gravy and the meat is tender. Season to taste
   before serving.

**17G CARBOHYDRATE PER SERVING • SERVE WITH CELERIAC MASH AND STEAMED
SAVOY CABBAGE AND PEAS**

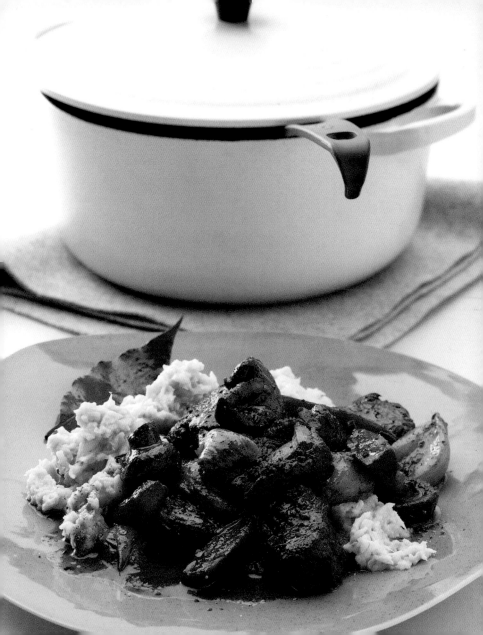

052

PAN-FRIED PORK WITH MINTY PEA PURÉE SERVES 2

1 tbsp olive oil
2 pork fillets, about 150g/5½oz each
chopped fresh parsley, to garnish

MINTY PEA PURÉE:
200g/7oz/1¼ cups frozen peas
2 tbsp chopped fresh mint
1 tbsp olive oil
2 tbsp reduced-fat crème fraîche
2 tbsp hot water
salt and freshly ground black pepper

1   To make the pea purée, boil the peas until cooked. Drain and transfer to a
    blender with the mint, olive oil, crème fraîche and hot water and purée until
    smooth. Season to taste and keep warm.

2   Heat the oil in a frying pan. Cook the pork for 4–5 minutes each side, then season
    well. Place the pea purée in a mound in the centre of each plate and top with the
    pork, then garnish with parsley.

10G CARBOHYDRATE PER SERVING • SERVE WITH STEAMED CARROTS

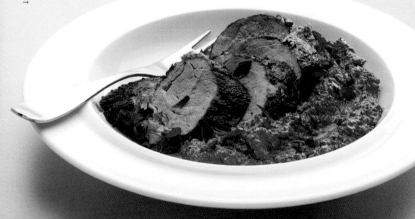

053

SPICED PORK WITH CORIANDER HOUMOUS SERVES 2

2 tbsp olive oil

1 tsp sweet paprika

1 tbsp chopped fresh rosemary

2 pork chops, about 175g/6oz each,
  fat trimmed

salt and freshly ground black pepper

CORIANDER HOUMOUS:

6 tbsp houmous

2 tbsp reduced-fat crème fraîche

2 tbsp chopped fresh coriander/cilantro

1   Mix together the oil, paprika and rosemary in a shallow dish. Season well. Add
    the pork and turn to coat in the marinade. Cover with cling film/plastic wrap and
    leave to marinate in the refrigerator for at least 1 hour.

2   Preheat the grill/broiler to its highest setting and line the grill/broiler pan with foil.
    Grill/broil the chops for 5–7 minutes each side, or until cooked through.

3   Meanwhile, mix together the houmous, crème fraîche and coriander/cilantro.
    Season and serve with the pork chops.

7.5G CARBOHYDRATE PER SERVING • SERVE WITH STEAMED COURGETTES/ZUCCHINI

MAIN MEALS – MEAT

054

SPICY MEATBALLS IN TOMATO SAUCE SERVES 2

300g/10½oz/1¼ cups lean minced/
  ground pork
1 onion, grated
1 tsp ground cumin
1 tsp paprika
1 large clove garlic, crushed
1 egg, beaten
salt and freshly ground black pepper

TOMATO SAUCE:
1 tbsp extra-virgin olive oil
2 cloves garlic, chopped
½ tsp dried crushed chilli flakes
400ml/14fl oz/1⅔ cups passata
1 bay leaf
2 tsp tomato purée/paste
2 tsp chopped fresh coriander/cilantro,
  to serve

1 Put the pork, onion, ground cumin, paprika, garlic and egg in a bowl and mix well until combined. Season with salt and pepper and refrigerate for 30 minutes.

2 Meanwhile, make the tomato sauce. Heat the olive oil in a large frying pan and fry the garlic and chillies for 1 minute.

3 Add the passata, bay leaf and tomato purée/paste, stir well, and cook over a medium-low heat, half-covered, for 5 minutes.

4 Remove the meatball mixture from the refrigerator and form into walnut-size balls. Place them in the sauce and cook, half-covered, over a medium-low heat for 15–20 minutes until they are cooked through. Sprinkle with coriander/cilantro before serving.

10G CARBOHYDRATE PER SERVING • SERVE WITH A SMALL WHOLEMEAL/ WHOLE-WHEAT PITTA BREAD AND A MIXED LEAF SALAD

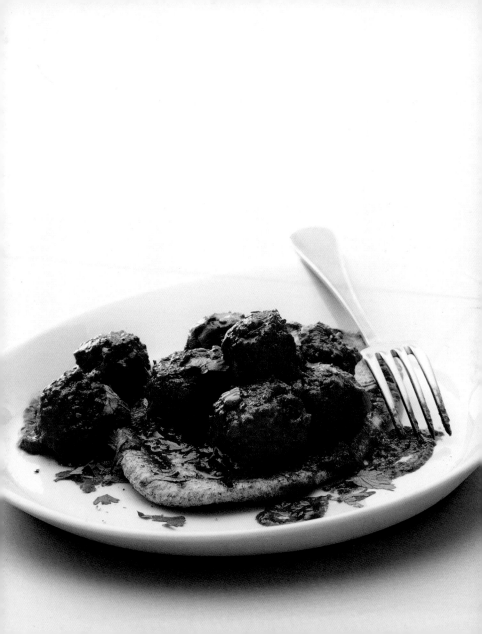

055

CHICKEN ESCALOPE WITH
MANGO SALSA SERVES 2

2 skinless chicken breasts, about
   150g/5½oz each
½ tsp lemon juice
salt and freshly ground black pepper
olive oil, for brushing

MANGO SALSA:
1 small mango, pitted and diced
¼ red onion, finely diced
juice of ½ lime
½ red chilli, seeded and finely chopped
2 tbsp torn fresh basil

1   To make the salsa, mix together the mango, red onion, lime juice, red chilli and
basil leaves. Season with salt and stir to combine.

2   Put the chicken breasts between two sheets of cling film/plastic wrap and flatten
with the end of a rolling pin. Squeeze over a little lemon juice and season.

3   Heat a griddle pan and brush with oil. Griddle the chicken for about 3–4 minutes
on each side, depending on the thickness of the fillet, until cooked through. Serve
with the mango salsa.

**8G CARBOHYDRATE PER SERVING • SERVE WITH CAULIFLOWER 'RICE' AND
A GREEN SALAD**

MAIN MEALS – POULTRY

Recipe pictured on page 71 (top right)

056

MALAY CHICKEN CURRY SERVES 2

1 tbsp olive oil
1 onion, grated
4 skinless chicken thighs
2 tsp grated fresh ginger
2 large cloves garlic, crushed
1 stick lemongrass, peeled and crushed
   using the back of a knife
2 tsp ground cumin
2 tsp ground coriander
1 tsp ground turmeric
1 cinnamon stick
2 cloves

2 cardamom pods, split
1/2 tsp hot chilli powder
1 bird's eye chilli, finely chopped
150ml/5fl oz/2/3 cup reduced-fat
   coconut milk
100ml/31/2fl oz/1/2 cup vegetable stock
   (see page 23)
salt
juice of 1/2 lime
2 tbsp chopped fresh coriander/cilantro,
   to garnish

1   Heat the oil in a large saucepan. Add the onion and fry, half-covered, for
    5 minutes. Add the chicken thighs and brown for about 5 minutes, turning until
    golden all over. Remove the chicken from the pan.
2   Add the ginger, garlic, lemongrass, spices and fresh chilli and cook for 2 minutes,
    stirring continuously. Add 3 tablespoons of water and cook for a further 2 minutes.
3   Return the chicken to the pan with the coconut milk, stock and a little salt. Bring
    to the boil, then reduce the heat and simmer, half-covered, for 40 minutes, stirring
    occasionally, until the chicken is cooked through and the sauce has reduced
    and thickened.
4   Stir in the lime juice and heat through, then serve sprinkled with coriander/cilantro.

8G CARBOHYDRATE PER SERVING • SERVE WITH A SMALL BOWL OF BROWN
BASMATI RICE

057

CHICKEN WITH LEMON QUINOA

SERVES 2

2 skinless chicken breasts, about
  150g/5½oz each
olive oil, for brushing
2 tsp crushed coriander seeds
salt and freshly ground black pepper

LEMON QUINOA:
55g/2oz/¼ cup quinoa
hot vegetable stock (see page 23),
  to cover
juice and finely grated zest of ½ lemon
2 tbsp chopped fresh thyme

1 Put the quinoa in a saucepan and cover with stock until it is about 1cm/½in
    above the level of the quinoa. Bring to the boil, reduce the heat, cover and
    simmer for about 10 minutes until the stock has been absorbed and the grains
    are tender. Leave to stand, covered, for 5 minutes, then fluff up with a fork.

2 Preheat the grill/broiler to high and line the grill/broiler pan with foil. Put the
    quinoa in a bowl and stir in the lemon juice, zest and thyme. Stir well to combine
    and season to taste.

3 Arrange the chicken in the grill/broiler pan, brush with oil, sprinkle with the
    coriander seeds and season. Grill/broil for 5–6 minutes each side until cooked
    through and there is no trace of pink.

4 Divide the quinoa between two plates and top with the chicken breasts.

19G CARBOHYDRATE • SERVE WITH GRILLED/BROILED FENNEL

058

PROSCIUTTO-WRAPPED CHICKEN WITH MOZZARELLA SERVES 2

6 slices prosciutto

2 skinless chicken breasts, about
   150g/5½oz each

90g/3¼oz mozzarella, cut into 6 slices

4 basil leaves

1 tbsp olive oil

½ tsp lemon juice

salt and freshly ground black pepper

1 Preheat the oven to 200°C/400°F/Gas 6. Arrange 2 slices of prosciutto slightly overlapping on a plate. Place a chicken breast in the middle of the prosciutto slices and top with 3 slices mozzarella. Place 2 basil leaves on the mozzarella and sprinkle with a little olive oil. Season well.

2 Wrap the prosciutto around the chicken and filling, then place a third slice of prosciutto over the top of the parcel lengthways and tuck the ends in underneath. Repeat to make another parcel.

3 Brush a roasting pan with oil, place the chicken parcels in the pan and cover with foil. Roast for 10 minutes, remove the foil and cook for another 15 minutes or until the chicken is cooked through and there is no trace of pink.

4 Squeeze over a little lemon juice before serving.

1G CARBOHYDRATE PER SERVING • SERVE WITH QUINOA TABBOULEH (SEE PAGE 43)

MAIN MEALS – POULTRY

059

SPANISH CHICKEN CASSEROLE

SERVES 2

4 chicken thighs
soy flour, for dusting
salt and freshly ground black pepper
1½ tbsp olive oil
1 large red onion, sliced
1 small orange pepper, seeded and
  sliced
2 large cloves garlic, chopped

100ml/3½fl oz/½ cup chicken stock
  (see page 22)
100ml/3½fl oz/½ cup dry sherry
1 bay leaf
zest and juice of ½ orange
½ tsp smoked paprika
1 tsp Worcestershire sauce
40g/1½oz/¼ cup black olives

1 Dust the chicken in seasoned flour. Heat ½ tbsp of the oil in a casserole dish, add
   the chicken and cook for 7 minutes, turning halfway, until golden. Remove from
   the pan and keep warm.

2 Pour away any oil in the pan and heat the remaining oil. Add the onion and fry,
   covered, for 5 minutes. Add the pepper and garlic and cook, covered, for another
   5 minutes. Return the chicken to the pan.

3 Add the stock, sherry, bay leaf, orange zest and juice, paprika, Worcestershire
   sauce and olives, then bring to the boil. Reduce the heat and simmer, half-covered,
   for 30–35 minutes until the chicken is cooked through and the sauce has reduced
   and thickened.

11G CARBOHYDRATE PER SERVING • SERVE WITH BRAISED LEEKS

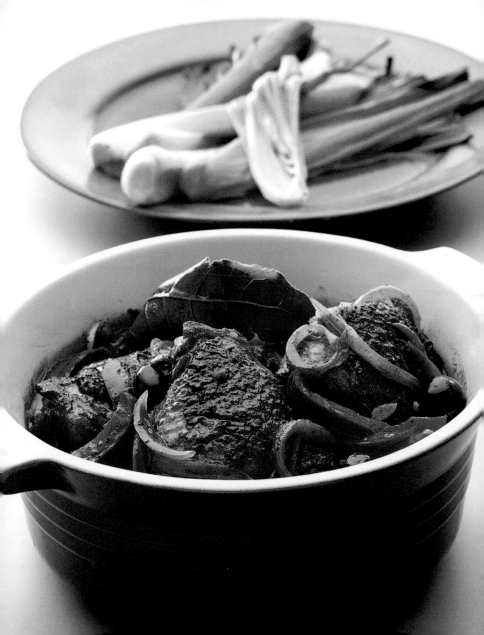

060

CHILLI CHICKEN WITH
BUTTERNUT SQUASH MASH SERVES 2

2 skinless chicken breasts, about
   150g/5½oz each
2 tbsp olive oil
4 tsp harissa paste
350g/12oz/2 cups peeled and cubed
   butternut squash (about 750g/1lb 10oz
   whole squash)

2 cloves garlic, left whole but peeled
1 tbsp reduced-fat mayonnaise
salt and freshly ground black pepper
1 tbsp chopped fresh coriander/cilantro,
   to garnish

1   Cut shallow slashes in each chicken breast, brush with half of the oil and coat
    both sides in the harissa paste. Season well and chill, covered, for 30 minutes.
    Preheat the oven to 220°C/425°F/Gas 7.
2   Put the chicken in a roasting pan and roast for about 30 minutes.
3   Meanwhile, put the squash and garlic in a saucepan, cover with water and bring
    to the boil. Cook for 10 minutes, drain well, and add the mayonnaise and the
    remaining olive oil. Season well and mash until smooth.
4   Divide the squash between two plates and top with the chicken. Sprinkle with
    coriander/cilantro before serving.

17G CARBOHYDRATE PER SERVING • SERVE WITH STEAMED BROCCOLI

061

TAPENADE CHICKEN SERVES 2

a little oil for roasting

2 skinless chicken breasts, about
150g/5½oz each

TAPENADE:

100g/3½oz/⅔ cup pitted green olives,
rinsed if in brine

1 clove garlic, crushed

1 tbsp capers, rinsed

1 large handful of parsley leaves

1 tbsp extra-virgin olive oil

freshly ground black pepper

1 To make the tapenade, put the olives, garlic, capers, parsley and oil in a food processor and blend until finely chopped. Season to taste with pepper.

2 Preheat the oven to 200°C/400°F/Gas 6. Lightly oil a roasting pan. Arrange the chicken breasts in the pan and cover each one with the tapenade.

3 Cover the pan with foil and roast for 10 minutes, then remove the foil and cook for another 10 minutes or until the chicken is cooked through and there is no trace of pink.

5.5G CARBOHYDRATE PER SERVING • SERVE WITH SWISS CHARD SAUTÉED WITH GARLIC AND LEMON ZEST

062

GINGER CHICKEN WITH SAUTÉED SPINACH SERVES 2

2 tbsp olive oil

280g/10oz chicken, cut into bite-size
pieces

3 tomatoes, seeded and diced

1 clove garlic, chopped

1cm/½in piece fresh ginger, peeled
and grated

1 tsp toasted sesame oil

140g/5oz/2½ cups baby spinach leaves

1 tbsp lemon juice

salt and freshly ground black pepper

1   Heat half the olive oil in a sauté pan. Add the chicken and fry for 5 minutes until
     sealed and golden on all sides. Stir in the tomatoes, garlic and ginger and cook
     for 3 minutes.

2   Add 2 tablespoons of water and cook over a medium-low heat until reduced
     and the chicken is cooked through. Season to taste, remove the mixture from the
     pan and keep warm.

3   Wipe the pan and add the remaining olive oil and sesame oil. Heat the oils,
     then add the spinach and lemon juice and season. Cook the spinach, stirring
     continuously, for 2–3 minutes until wilted.

4   Divide the spinach between 2 serving plates and top with the chicken mixture.

4.5G CARBOHYDRATE PER SERVING • SERVE WITH CHICKPEA MASH (SEE PAGE 127)

063

INDIAN TURKEY WITH SPINACH

SERVES 2

1 tbsp olive oil
1 onion, chopped
2 cloves garlic, chopped
225g/8oz/1 cup minced/ground turkey
3 tbsp curry paste of your choice
200g/7oz/1 cup canned chopped
  tomatoes

150ml/5fl oz/²/₃ cup chicken stock
  (see page 22)
70g/2¹/₂oz/¹/₃ cup canned chickpeas/
  garbanzo beans, rinsed
100g/3¹/₂oz/1³/₄ cups fresh spinach
salt and freshly ground black pepper

1   Heat the oil in a saucepan and cook the onion, half-covered, for 8 minutes. Add
    the garlic and turkey and cook over a medium heat for 5 minutes. Stir in the curry
    paste and cook for another minute.
2   Stir in the tomatoes, stock and chickpeas/garbanzo beans and cook, half-covered,
    for 15–20 minutes until the sauce has reduced and thickened. Add the spinach
    and heat through for 3 minutes until wilted. Season to taste before serving.

11G CARBOHYDRATE PER SERVING • SERVE WITH A SMALL BOWL OF BROWN
BASMATI RICE

064

TURKEY & MANGO STIR-FRY SERVES 2

1 tbsp groundnut or sunflower oil

250g/9oz turkey breasts, cut into strips

1 clove garlic, chopped

1 bird's eye chilli, seeded and finely
  chopped

juice of 1 lime

1 tbsp Thai fish sauce

2 spring onions/scallions, sliced on
  the diagonal

2 small heads pak choi/bok choy,
  sliced

1 small mango, pitted and sliced

chopped fresh coriander/cilantro,
  to garnish

1   Heat the oil in a wok. When hot, add the turkey and stir-fry for 6–8 minutes or until
    cooked through. Transfer to a plate and keep warm.
2   Add the garlic, chilli, lime juice, fish sauce, spring onions/scallions and pak choi/
    bok choy to the wok and stir-fry for a further 2–3 minutes. Return the turkey to
    the wok with the mango and stir to combine. Serve sprinkled with chopped fresh
    coriander/cilantro.

17G CARBOHYDRATE PER SERVING • SERVE WITH CAULIFLOWER 'RICE'

MAIN MEALS – POULTRY

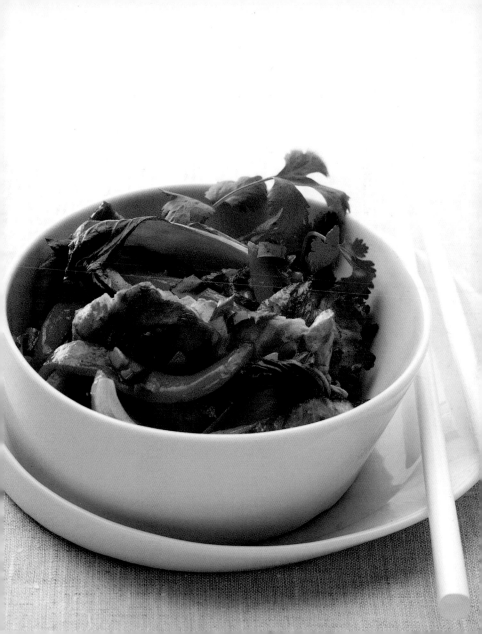

065

BAKED LEMON COD WITH
SALSA VERDE SERVES 2

2 thick cod fillets, about 200g/7oz each
olive oil, for brushing
4 thin slices lemon
salt and freshly ground black pepper

SALSA VERDE:
3 tbsp olive oil
1 clove garlic, crushed
3 tbsp chopped fresh parsley
2 tbsp chopped fresh mint
juice of ½ lemon

1   Preheat the oven to 200°C/400°F/Gas 6. Rinse and dry each cod fillet and brush
    with olive oil. Place each fillet on a piece of foil that is large enough to cover
    the fish and make a parcel. Top each fillet with two slices of lemon and season.
    Fold over the foil to encase the fish and bake for 20 minutes or until just cooked
    and opaque.

2   Meanwhile, to make the salsa verde, put the olive oil, garlic, parsley, mint and
    lemon juice in a blender and process until finely chopped. Season to taste.

3   Carefully unfold each parcel and place on serving plates. Place a spoonful of
    salsa by the side of each piece of fish before serving.

1G CARBOHYDRATE PER SERVING • SERVE WITH A SMALL BOWL OF BROWN RICE
MIXED WITH WILD RICE

MAIN MEALS – FISH & SEAFOOD

Recipe pictured on page 71 (bottom left)

066

MAPLE-GLAZED TUNA <small>SERVES 2</small>

4 tsp soy sauce

2 tbsp olive oil

1 tsp grated fresh ginger

1 clove garlic, crushed

1 tsp maple syrup

2 tuna steaks, about 125g/4½oz each

salt and freshly ground black pepper

1   Mix together the soy sauce, oil, ginger, garlic and maple syrup. Season and add the tuna steaks. Spoon over the marinade to coat the fish, cover and leave to marinate in the refrigerator for about 1 hour.

2   Preheat the grill/broiler to high and line the grill/broiler pan with foil. Grill/broil the tuna for about 2 minutes each side, occasionally spooning the marinade over the fish.

4G CARBOHYDRATE PER SERVING • SERVE WITH A SMALL BOWL OF WHOLE-WHEAT NOODLES AND SPINACH SPRINKLED WITH TOASTED SESAME SEEDS

MAIN MEALS – FISH & SEAFOOD

067

SPICY MOROCCAN TUNA SERVES 2

1 tsp cumin seeds

1 tsp caraway seeds

1½ tbsp olive oil

2 cloves garlic, sliced

1 bird's eye chilli, seeded and finely
  chopped

100ml/3½fl oz/½ cup water

juice of ½ lemon

4 tbsp tomato purée/paste

2 tuna steaks, about 140g/5oz each

salt

chopped fresh coriander/cilantro

1 Grind the cumin and caraway seeds in a pestle and mortar. Heat the oil in
   a sauté pan and fry the garlic, spices and chilli for 1 minute. Add the water, lemon
   juice and tomato purée/paste and simmer for 5 minutes.

2 Add the tuna and spoon over the sauce, then cook for 5–8 minutes, depending
   on the thickness of the fish. Season with salt and sprinkle with coriander/cilantro.

9G CARBOHYDRATE PER SERVING • SERVE WITH QUINOA TABBOULEH (SEE PAGE 43)

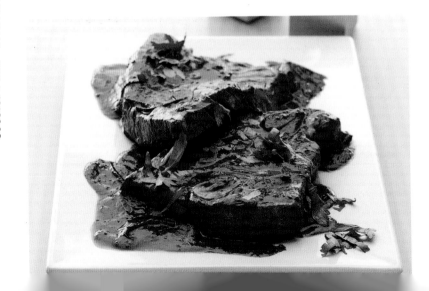

068

RED SNAPPER WITH ROMESCO SAUCE SERVES 2

4 red snapper fillets, about 175g/6oz
  each
olive oil, for brushing
salt and freshly ground black pepper

ROMESCO SAUCE:
30g/1oz/¼ cup chopped almonds
3 tomatoes, peeled, seeded and diced
2 tbsp olive oil
1 small clove garlic, sliced
2 tsp red wine vinegar
handful of fresh flat-leaf parsley
½ tsp paprika

1   Preheat the grill/broiler to high and line the grill/broiler pan with foil.
2   To make the sauce, lightly toast the almonds in a dry frying pan until golden. Put
    in a food processor or blender with the rest of the sauce ingredients and blitz until
    very finely chopped and a sauce consistency; season.
3   Lightly brush the red snapper with oil and grill/broil for about 3 minutes each side,
    then season before serving with the sauce.

3G CARBOHYDRATE PER SERVING • SERVE WITH CHICKPEA MASH (SEE PAGE 127)

MAIN MEALS – FISH & SEAFOOD

069

CRISP SEA BASS WITH JAPANESE PICKLED VEGETABLES SERVES 2

4 sea bass fillets
2 tbsp lime juice
1 tsp rice vinegar
1 small clove garlic, crushed
1 bird's eye chilli, seeded and finely chopped
salt
fresh basil leaves, to garnish

PICKLED VEGETABLES:
1 carrot, finely shredded
5cm/2in piece cucumber, seeds scooped out and finely shredded
1 spring onion/scallion, finely shredded
2 tbsp rice vinegar

HOT CHILLI DIP:
2 tbsp reduced-fat mayonnaise
1½ tsp Thai red curry paste
1 tbsp olive oil

MAIN MEALS – FISH & SEAFOOD

1   Place the sea bass, skin-side down, in a shallow dish. Mix together the lime juice, vinegar, garlic and chilli. Pour the mixture over the sea bass and season with salt. Cover and leave in the refrigerator for 30 minutes.

2   To make the pickled vegetables, put the carrot, cucumber and spring onion/scallion in a small bowl. Pour over the vinegar and mix together.

3   To make the hot chilli dip, mix together the mayonnaise, Thai red curry paste and olive oil in a small bowl.

4   Preheat the grill/broiler to high and line the grill/broiler pan with foil. Place the sea bass, skin-side up, in the pan and brush with the marinade. Grill/broil for about 3–4 minutes until the skin becomes crisp.

5   Drain the pickled vegetables. Serve the sea bass with the vegetables and dip, sprinkled with fresh basil.

9G CARBOHYDRATE PER SERVING • SERVE WITH A SMALL BOWL OF SOBA NOODLES

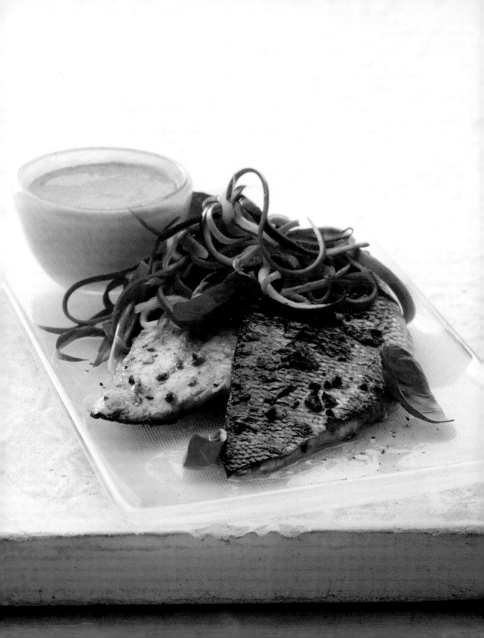

070

POACHED SALMON IN SHALLOT SAUCE SERVES 2

2 tsp olive oil
1 leek, finely sliced
1 shallot, diced
1 bay leaf
200ml/7fl oz/1 cup dry white wine

150ml/5fl oz/²/₃ cup fish stock
2 salmon fillets, about 125g/4¹/₂oz each
15g/¹/₂oz/1 tbsp butter
salt and freshly ground black pepper

1   Heat the oil in a large sauté pan and fry the leek, shallot and bay leaf over a
    medium heat for 4 minutes, stirring frequently.
2   Increase the heat and add the wine, then cook at a rolling boil until the wine has
    reduced by half.
3   Reduce the heat, add the stock and salmon, then cover with the lid and poach
    the fish for 6–8 minutes, turning halfway, until cooked. Remove the salmon and
    keep warm.
4   Add the butter to the pan and heat though, stirring continuously, until the butter
    has melted and the stock has reduced to form a sauce. Remove the bay leaf and
    season to taste. Put the salmon on serving plates and spoon over the sauce.

4G CARBOHYDRATE PER SERVING • SERVE WITH CAULIFLOWER MASH

071

MARINATED SALMON IN LIME & GINGER SERVES 2

2 salmon fillets, about 125g/4½oz each
1 hot red chilli, sliced into rounds
juice of 1 lime
1 tbsp fresh orange juice
1cm/½in piece fresh ginger, peeled
  and grated

175g/6oz fine green beans
salt and freshly ground black pepper
1 spring onion/scallion, sliced on the
  diagonal, to garnish

1 Thinly slice each salmon fillet on the diagonal. Mix together the chilli, lime juice,
   orange juice and ginger in a shallow dish. Add the salmon slices and spoon over
   the marinade. Cover and marinate in the refrigerator for at least 1 hour.
2 Steam the green beans.
3 Meanwhile, heat a griddle pan until hot. Add the salmon slices and cook for
   1½ minutes until just cooked.
4 Divide the green beans between two serving plates. Heat the marinade through in
   a saucepan. Place the salmon on top of the beans and spoon over the marinade;
   season. Sprinkle with the spring onion/scallion before serving.

5G CARBOHYDRATE PER SERVING • SERVE WITH COURGETTE/ZUCCHINI 'NOODLES'

072

GLAZED SALMON WITH ASPARAGUS SERVES 2

2 salmon fillets, about 140g/5oz each
olive oil, for brushing
10 spears asparagus, ends trimmed
1 tbsp sesame seeds, toasted

MARINADE:
1 clove garlic, crushed
4 tbsp fresh apple juice
1 tbsp soy sauce
1 tbsp sunflower oil
1 tsp toasted sesame oil
salt and freshly ground black pepper

1   Mix together the ingredients for the marinade and season. Place the salmon in a shallow dish and pour the marinade over, turning the fish to ensure it is completely covered. Leave to marinate in the refrigerator, covered, for at least 1 hour, turning the fish occasionally.

2   Preheat the grill/broiler to high. Line the grill/broiler pan with foil and place the salmon on top. Brush the fish with the marinade and grill/broil for about 6 minutes, turning once, until just cooked.

3   Meanwhile, heat a griddle pan and brush with olive oil. Arrange the asparagus in the pan and cook for 3–4 minutes until tender.

4   Place the remaining marinade in a small saucepan and heat until thickened and reduced.

5   Arrange the asparagus on two plates, then top with the salmon. Spoon the marinade over the fish and sprinkle with the sesame seeds.

7G CARBOHYDRATE PER SERVING • SERVE WITH A SMALL BOWL OF QUINOA

MAIN MEALS – FISH & SEAFOOD

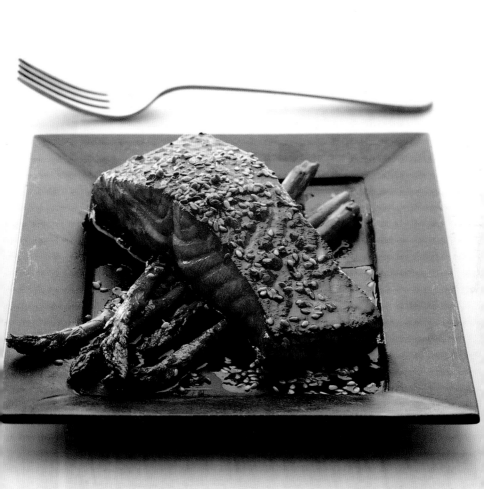

073

ORIENTAL FISH EN PAPILLOTE

SERVES 2

2 thick cod fillets, about 200g/7oz each
1 clove garlic, thinly sliced
2 thin slices fresh ginger, peeled and cut
   into matchsticks
2 small leeks, cut into thin strips
1 small carrot, cut into thin strips
¼ red pepper, cut into thin strips

2 tbsp lime juice
2 tsp light soy sauce
1 tbsp fresh apple juice
½ tsp sesame oil
salt and freshly ground black pepper
fresh coriander/cilantro, to garnish

1   Preheat the oven to 200°C/400°F/Gas 6. Place each cod fillet onto a piece of foil
    or baking parchment large enough to encase the fish. Arrange the garlic, ginger,
    leeks, carrot and pepper on top of each piece of cod.

2   Mix together the lime juice, soy sauce, apple juice and sesame oil, then spoon the
    mixture over the fish. Season to taste, then fold the foil or paper to make a loose
    parcel. Put the parcels on a baking sheet and bake for 15 minutes until the fish is
    just cooked. Serve garnished with sprigs of coriander/cilantro.

5G CARBOHYDRATE PER SERVING • SERVE WITH A SMALL BOWL OF QUINOA

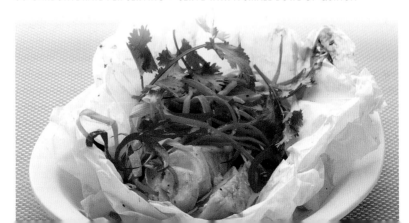

074

MONKFISH & VEGETABLE ROAST

SERVES 2

1 red pepper, seeded and sliced
1/2 fennel bulb, sliced
6 shallots, peeled and halved
olive oil, for brushing
2 skinless, boneless monkfish fillets,
   about 200g/7oz each
salt and freshly ground black pepper

BASIL OIL:
2½ tbsp extra-virgin olive oil
15g/½oz/¼ cup fresh basil
1 small clove garlic, crushed

1   Preheat the oven to 200°C/400°F/Gas 6. Put the red pepper, fennel and shallots in
    a large roasting pan and brush with oil. Roast for 15 minutes.
2   Meanwhile, heat a little oil in a frying pan over a medium-high heat. Add the fish
    and cook for 1–2 minutes each side until golden and sealed. Place the fish on top
    of the roasting vegetables and cook for a further 12–15 minutes.
3   To make the basil oil, gently heat the olive oil until just warm. Transfer the oil to a
    blender with the basil and garlic and purée; season.
4   Arrange the vegetables on a plate, top with the fish and drizzle over the basil oil.
    Season to taste.

**8G CARBOHYDRATE PER SERVING • SERVE WITH STEAMED GREEN VEGETABLES AND
CHICKPEA MASH (SEE PAGE 127)**

MAIN MEALS – FISH & SEAFOOD

075

THAI-STYLE MUSSELS SERVES 2

1 tbsp olive oil

2 shallots, chopped

2 cloves garlic, chopped

1 stick lemongrass, peeled and finely chopped

2 kaffir lime leaves

100ml/3½fl oz/½ cup dry white wine

75ml/2½fl oz/⅓ cup fish stock

juice of ½ lime

2 tbsp Thai tom yam paste

750g/1lb 10oz mussels, scrubbed and thoroughly rinsed

1 tbsp chopped fresh coriander/cilantro, to garnish

1   Heat the oil in a large, deep saucepan and cook the shallots for 5 minutes until softened. Add the garlic, lemongrass and kaffir lime leaves and cook for another minute.

2   Pour in the wine, fish stock and lime juice and bring to the boil. Stir in the tom yam paste, reduce the heat and simmer for 5 minutes until reduced.

3   Add the mussels, cover, and simmer over a medium heat for 5 minutes, shaking the pan occasionally, until the mussels have opened. Discard any mussels that have not opened. Serve immediately, sprinkled with coriander/cilantro.

25G CARBOHYDRATE PER SERVING • SERVE WITH A SMALL BOWL OF BROWN RICE

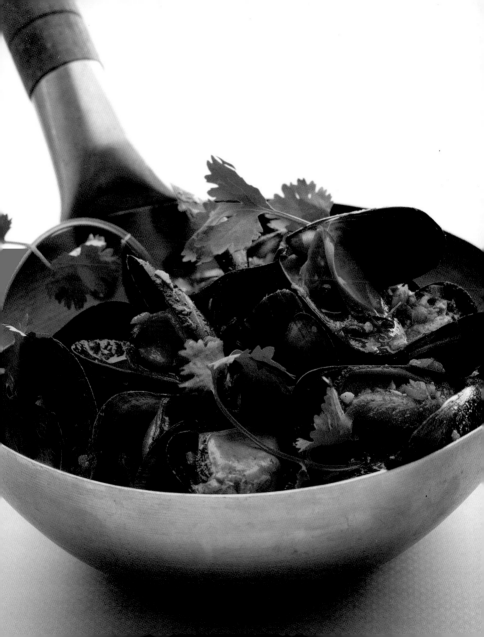

076

SEAFOOD STEW WITH ROUILLE

SERVES 2

1 tbsp olive oil

1 onion, finely sliced

1 tsp fennel seeds

150ml/5fl oz/²⁄₃ cup dry white wine

200g/7oz/1 cup canned chopped
  tomatoes

300g/10¹⁄₂oz cod fillets, skinned and cut
  into large bite-size pieces

150g/5¹⁄₂oz/1 cup mixed cooked
  seafood, such as prawns, squid
  and mussels

1 tbsp chopped fresh coriander/cilantro,
  to garnish

ROUILLE:

1 clove garlic, crushed

3 tbsp reduced-fat mayonnaise

¹⁄₂ tsp harissa paste

salt and freshly ground black pepper

MAIN MEALS – FISH & SEAFOOD

1   To make the rouille, mix together the garlic, mayonnaise and harissa in a bowl.
    Season to taste and set aside.

2   Heat the oil in a large lidded saucepan and fry the onion for 8 minutes, half
    covered, stirring occasionally. Add the fennel seeds and cook for 1 minute.

3   Pour in the wine and tomatoes and bring to the boil, then reduce the heat and
    simmer, half-covered, for 8 minutes. Add the fish and cook for about 4 minutes,
    then add the seafood and heat through, occasionally stirring gently. Season.

4   Serve in large shallow bowls, topped with a spoonful of rouille and sprinkled
    with coriander/cilantro.

7G CARBOHYDRATE PER SERVING • SERVE WITH A MIXED LEAF SALAD SPRINKLED
WITH TOASTED SEEDS

077

CLAMS WITH GARLIC & CHILLI

SERVES 2

500g/1lb 2oz small fresh clams
1 tbsp olive oil
2 cloves garlic, finely chopped
1 red chilli, seeded and finely chopped

200ml/7fl oz/1 cup dry white wine
salt and freshly ground black pepper
1 tbsp chopped fresh parsley, to garnish
lemon wedges, to serve

1 Rinse the clams well, discarding any with broken or open shells. Put the clams
   in a large saucepan and just cover with water. Bring to the boil and cook for
   2 minutes. Drain the clams, reserving the cooking liquor, and discard any shells
   that remain closed.

2 Heat the oil in a large sauté pan and fry the garlic and chilli for 1 minute.
   Increase the heat, add the white wine and cook until reduced. Add a quarter
   of the reserved cooking liquor and cook for a few minutes. Season to taste.

3 Divide the clams between two shallow bowls. Pour the sauce over the clams
   and sprinkle with parsley. Serve with wedges of lemon to squeeze over.

8.5G CARBOHYDRATE PER SERVING • SERVE WITH A SMALL BOWL OF WHOLE-WHEAT
SPAGHETTI AND A GREEN LEAF SALAD

078

CALAMARI WITH TOMATOES & OLIVES SERVES 2

2 tbsp olive oil
1 large clove garlic, chopped
1 tsp dried oregano
¼ tsp dried crushed chilli flakes
200g/7oz/1 cup canned chopped
  tomatoes

100ml/3½fl oz/½ cup dry white wine
30g/1oz/2 tbsp small black olives
280g/10oz squid rings
1 tbsp lemon juice
salt and freshly ground black pepper
chopped fresh parsley, to garnish

1   Heat the oil in a sauté pan. Fry the garlic for 1 minute, then add the oregano,
    chilli, tomatoes and wine. Bring to the boil, then reduce the heat and simmer,
    half-covered, for 10–12 minutes until reduced and thickened.

2   Add the olives and squid and cook, half-covered, over a low heat for 30 minutes.

3   Season to taste and stir in the lemon juice. Serve sprinkled with parsley.

10G CARBOHYDRATE PER SERVING • SERVE WITH WHOLE-WHEAT PASTA

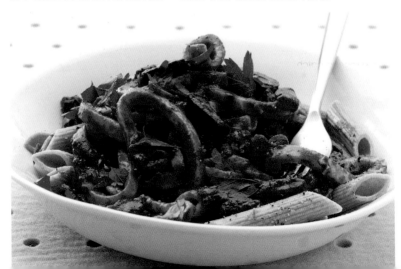

079

CARIBBEAN PRAWN BALLS WITH MANGO SAUCE SERVES 3

250g/9oz firm skinless white fish
125g/4½oz/⅔ cup medium cooked
   prawns/shrimp
½ tsp English mustard powder
1 shallot, roughly chopped
1 clove garlic, crushed
½ tsp cayenne pepper
juice of 1 lime
1 tsp dried thyme

sunflower oil, for frying
salt and freshly ground black pepper

MANGO SAUCE:
½ mango, pitted and flesh scooped
   out of the skin
1 tsp lemon juice
½ tsp dried chilli flakes

1   Put the fish, prawns/shrimp, mustard powder, shallot, garlic, cayenne pepper,
    lime juice and thyme in a food processor. Season well and process until a thick
    paste. Leave to chill, covered, for 30 minutes to allow the mixture to firm up.
2   Form the prawn/shrimp mixture into 12 balls each the size of a large walnut,
    then flatten the tops slightly. Pour enough oil to lightly cover the base of a large,
    heavy frying pan. Heat the oil and fry the balls in two batches for 2 minutes each
    side until lightly golden. Drain on paper towels and keep warm while you cook
    the second batch.
3   Meanwhile, put the mango, lemon juice and chilli flakes into a blender and
    process until puréed. Season with salt and pour into a small bowl.
4   Serve the prawn/shrimp balls with the sauce on the side.

8G CARBOHYDRATE PER SERVING • SERVE WITH CAULIFLOWER 'RICE'

080

MALAYSIAN-STYLE COCONUT PRAWNS SERVES 4

2 tsp groundnut or sunflower oil

½ red pepper, seeded and diced

1 small head pak choi/bok choy, stalks thinly sliced and leaves chopped

1 large clove garlic, chopped

½ tsp ground turmeric

2 tsp garam masala

1 tsp chilli powder

75ml/2½fl oz/⅓ cup hot vegetable stock (see page 23)

2 tbsp no-sugar smooth peanut butter

150ml/5fl oz/⅔ cup reduced-fat coconut milk

2 tsp soy sauce

150g/5½oz/¾ cup raw tiger prawns/ shrimp, peeled

1 spring onion/scallion, finely chopped on the diagonal

1 tsp sesame seeds, toasted

1 Heat the oil in a wok or large heavy frying pan. Add the red pepper, pak choi/bok choy stalks and garlic and stir-fry for 3 minutes. Add the turmeric, garam masala, chilli powder and pak choi/bok choy leaves and stir-fry for another 1 minute.

2 Mix together the hot stock and peanut butter until the latter has dissolved and add to the stir-fry with the coconut milk and soy sauce. Cook for 3 minutes or until reduced and thickened.

3 Add the prawns/shrimp to the coconut curry and cook for a further 3–5 minutes until cooked through.

4 Spoon into shallow bowls and sprinkle with the spring onion/scallion and toasted sesame seeds.

8.5G CARBOHYDRATE PER SERVING • SERVE WITH A SMALL BOWL OF WHOLE-WHEAT NOODLES

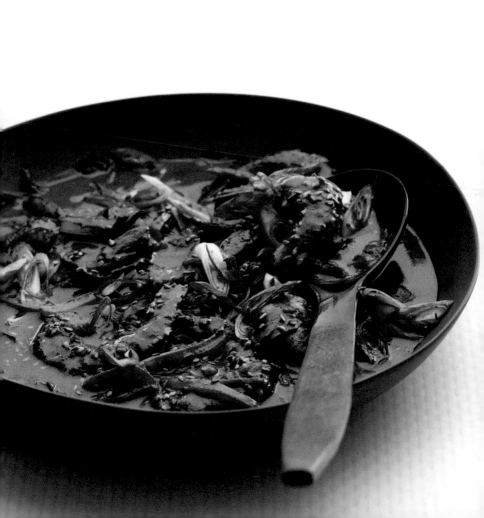

081

AUBERGINE, SMOKED
MOZZARELLA & BASIL ROLLS SERVES 2

1 aubergine/eggplant
2 tbsp olive oil, plus extra for drizzling
85g/3oz smoked mozzarella, cut into
    6 slices

1 vine-ripened tomato, cut into 6 slices
6 large basil leaves
salt and freshly ground black pepper
1 tsp balsamic vinegar, for drizzling

1   Cut the aubergine/eggplant lengthways into 6 thin slices and discard the two
    outermost slices.
2   Preheat the grill/broiler to medium-high and line the rack with foil. Place the
    aubergine/eggplant slices on the grill/broiler rack and brush with the oil. Grill/broil
    for 8–10 minutes until tender, turning once, and brushing with extra oil, if necessary.
3   Remove from the grill/broiler, then place a slice of mozzarella, a slice of tomato
    and a basil leaf in the middle of each aubergine/eggplant slice, season to taste.
    Fold the aubergine/eggplant over the filling and grill/broil, seam-side down, for
    3 minutes or until the mozzarella begins to melt. Serve drizzled with olive oil and
    balsamic vinegar.

**4G CARBOHYDRATE PER SERVING • SERVE WITH A MIXED LEAF SALAD SPRINKLED
WITH TOASTED SEEDS**

Recipe pictured on page 71 (bottom right)

082

OPEN 'LASAGNE' WITH PORCINI MUSHROOMS & OLIVES SERVES 2

40g/1½oz/¼ cup dried porcini mushrooms
2 tbsp olive oil
2 cloves garlic, chopped
1 tsp dried oregano
140g/5oz/1¼ cups field mushrooms, sliced
100ml/3½fl oz/½ cup dry white wine
3 tbsp canned chopped tomatoes

40g/1½oz/¼ cup small black olives
50g/1¾oz/½ cup drained and rinsed canned butter/lima beans
salt and freshly ground black pepper
2 courgettes/zucchini, cut into long, thin slices
30g/1oz/¼ cup Parmesan shavings
salt and freshly ground black pepper
basil leaves, to garnish

1. Place the porcini mushrooms in a bowl and cover with boiling water. Leave to soak for 15 minutes, then drain, rinse and pat dry.
2. Heat the oil in a large frying pan and sauté the porcini over a high heat for 5 minutes until they become slightly crisp around the edges. Add the garlic, oregano and field mushrooms and cook for another 5 minutes.
3. Pour in the wine and tomatoes. Bring to the boil, then reduce the heat and simmer for 5 minutes until reduced and thickened. Add the olives and beans and cook for 2 more minutes. Season to taste.
4. Meanwhile, steam the courgettes/zucchini until just tender.
5. To serve, spoon the mushroom sauce onto each plate. Sprinkle with some of the Parmesan, then top with the slices of courgette/zucchini. Sprinkle with more Parmesan and top with the basil.

16G CARBOHYDRATE PER SERVING • SERVE WITH A GREEN SALAD

083

ROASTED VEGETABLES WITH PESTO DRESSING SERVES 2

2 tbsp olive oil

1 tbsp balsamic vinegar

2 sprigs fresh rosemary

1 red pepper, seeded and quartered

1 courgette/zucchini, sliced lengthways

2 red onions, quartered

1 fennel bulb, sliced into thin wedges

8 tomatoes on the vine

1 bulb garlic, unpeeled with top sliced off

10 black olives

Parmesan shavings, to serve

PESTO DRESSING:

1 tbsp good-quality ready-made pesto

1 tbsp extra-virgin olive oil

1 tbsp hot water

1   Mix together the olive oil, vinegar and rosemary in a large shallow dish.

2   Place the red pepper, courgette/zucchini, red onions, fennel, tomatoes and garlic in the dish and toss them in the marinade. Leave to marinate for at least 1 hour. Meanwhile, preheat the oven to 200°C/400°F/Gas 6.

3   Put the vegetables (except the tomatoes), garlic and marinade in a roasting pan. Roast for 25 minutes, turning occasionally, then remove the rosemary. Add the tomatoes and olives, then return to the oven and cook for another 10–15 minutes until the vegetables are tender and slightly blackened at the edges.

4   Meanwhile, mix together the ingredients for the pesto dressing. Arrange the roasted vegetables on two plates and drizzle with a little dressing. Top with the Parmesan shavings to serve.

21G CARBOHYDRATE PER SERVING • SERVE WITH A SMALL GRIDDLED WHOLEMEAL/ WHOLE-WHEAT PITTA BREAD AND A GREEN SALAD

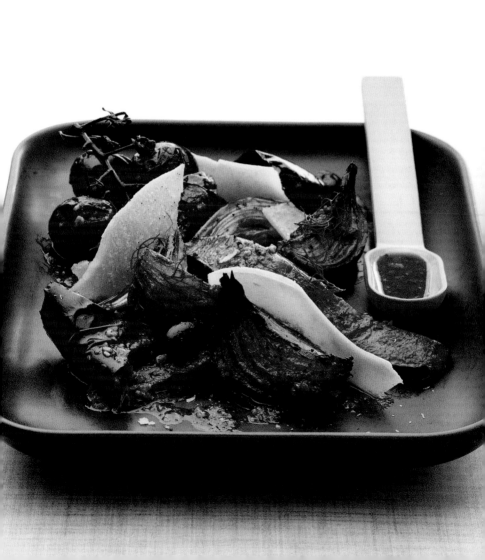

084

PEPPER & HALLOUMI KEBABS

SERVES 2 (MAKES 4 KEBABS)

2 small courgettes/zucchini, each cut
   into 4 chunks
8 cherry tomatoes
1 small orange pepper, seeded and cut
   into 8 chunks
140g/5oz halloumi cheese, cut into
   16 cubes
1 red onion, cut into 8 wedges

FOR THE MARINADE:
3 tbsp olive oil
2 tbsp balsamic vinegar
1 clove garlic, chopped
3 tbsp fresh orange juice
handful of chopped mixed herbs, such
   as oregano, marjoram and chives

MAIN MEALS – VEGETARIAN

1   Mix together the ingredients for the marinade in a shallow dish.
2   Arrange the vegetables and halloumi on 4 skewers (if using wooden skewers soak
    them in water for about 15 minutes beforehand to prevent them burning): thread
    2 pieces of courgette/zucchini, 2 cherry tomatoes, 2 pieces of pepper, 4 cubes
    of halloumi and 2 wedges of onion onto each skewer. Place the kebabs in the
    marinade, and turn to coat, then cover and marinate in the refrigerator for 1 hour.
3   Preheat the grill/broiler to high and line the grill/broiler pan with foil. Place the
    kebabs under the grill/broiler, spoon over the marinade, and cook for about
    8–10 minutes, turning occasionally, until tender and browned. Spoon over more
    marinade if the kebabs look dry.

13G CARBOHYDRATE PER SERVING • SERVE WITH A SMALL BOWL OF
WHOLE-WHEAT COUSCOUS

Recipe pictured on page 144

085

CREAMY BROCCOLI & CAULIFLOWER CHEESE SERVES 2

175g/6oz broccoli, cut into small florets
150g/5½oz cauliflower, cut into small
  florets
15g/½oz/1 tbsp butter
1½ tbsp soy flour

350ml/12fl oz/1½ cups milk, warmed
2 tsp Dijon mustard
70g/2½oz/⅔ cup grated mature
  Cheddar
salt and freshly ground black pepper

1   Steam the broccoli and cauliflower for 5 minutes until just cooked.
2   Meanwhile, make the cheese sauce. Melt the butter in a heavy saucepan.
    Stir in the flour and cook for about 2 minutes, stirring continuously, until it forms
    a thick light brown paste. Remove from the heat and gradually add the warm
    milk, whisking well with a balloon whisk after each addition. Continue to whisk
    to make a smooth, creamy sauce.
3   Return the white sauce to the heat and add the mustard. Cook for about
    10 minutes until the sauce has thickened. Mix in two-thirds of the cheese and
    stir well until it has melted. Season to taste. Pour the sauce over the vegetables
    in the dish and mix gently until combined.
4   Preheat the grill/broiler to high. Sprinkle the dish with the remaining cheese,
    then grill/broil for 5–10 minutes until the cheese is bubbling and golden.

13.5G CARBOHYDRATE PER SERVING • SERVE WITH PEAS

086

THAI GREEN VEGETABLE CURRY

SERVES 2

2 tsp sunflower oil

200ml/7fl oz/1 cup reduced-fat
  coconut milk

150ml/5fl oz/²⁄₃ cup vegetable stock
  (see page 23)

115g/4oz/1 cup small broccoli florets

1 corn on the cob, husk removed, sliced
  into 2cm/³⁄₄in pieces

1 small red pepper, seeded and sliced

55g/2oz/1 cup fresh spinach leaves,
  shredded

salt and freshly ground black pepper

1 tbsp chopped fresh coriander/cilantro,
  to garnish

SPICE PASTE:

3 green chillies, seeded and chopped

1 stick lemongrass, peeled and finely
  chopped

1 shallot, sliced

juice and zest of 1 lime

1 clove garlic, chopped

1 tsp ground coriander

1 tsp ground cumin

1cm/¹⁄₂in piece fresh ginger, peeled
  and grated

2 tbsp chopped fresh coriander/cilantro

1   Place all the ingredients for the spice paste in a food processor and blend to
    a coarse paste.

2   Heat the oil in a large saucepan and fry the spice paste for 1 minute, stirring.
    Add the coconut milk and stock and bring to the boil. Reduce the heat and
    simmer for 10 minutes until reduced.

3   Add the broccoli, corn and red pepper and cook for 3 minutes, then add the
    spinach and cook for another 2 minutes until the vegetables are just tender.

4   Season to taste and sprinkle with coriander/cilantro before serving.

11G CARBOHYDRATE PER SERVING • SERVE WITH A SMALL BOWL OF BROWN RICE

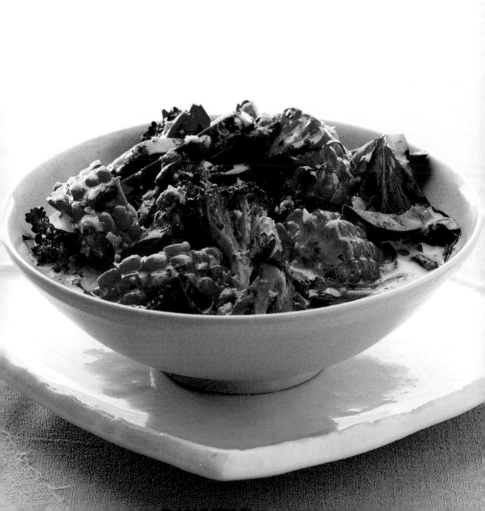

087

SPRING VEGETABLE STIR-FRY WITH CASHEWS SERVES 2

½ tbsp groundnut or vegetable oil
splash of toasted sesame oil
175g/6oz/1½ cups broccoli florets
2 spring onions/scallions, sliced on the
   diagonal
85g/3oz fine green beans, trimmed
2 heads pak choi/bok choy, sliced
   in half

1 clove garlic, chopped
1cm/½in piece fresh ginger, peeled
   and finely chopped
3 tbsp fresh apple juice
2 tsp soy sauce
70g/2½oz/⅔ cup unsalted cashew nuts,
   toasted
basil leaves, to garnish

1   Heat a frying pan or wok and add both the groundnut and sesame oil. Add the
   broccoli, spring onions/scallions and green beans. Stir-fry, tossing the vegetables
   continuously, for 5 minutes.

2   Add the pak choi/bok choy, garlic and ginger and stir fry for another 1 minute.
   Pour in the apple juice and soy sauce and cook for 1–2 minutes (add a little water
   if the stir-fry appears too dry). Sprinkle with cashew nuts and basil.

**13G CARBOHYDRATE PER SERVING •
SERVE WITH CAULIFLOWER 'RICE'**

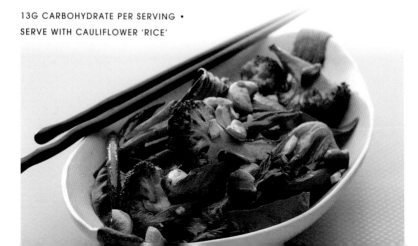

088

MIXED NUT ROAST SERVES 2

1 tbsp olive oil
1 onion, finely chopped
1 carrot, grated
1 small parsnip, grated
1 tsp dried mixed herbs
1 tsp dried thyme
50g/1¾oz/½ cup unsalted peanuts
50g/1¾oz/½ cup hazelnuts

1 slice wholemeal/whole-wheat bread,
  crusts removed
1 tbsp sunflower seeds
2 tsp vegetarian Worcestershire sauce
1 tsp bouillon powder (stock)
1 egg, beaten
salt and freshly ground black pepper

1   Preheat the oven to 200°C/400°F/Gas 6. Heat the oil in a saucepan, add the
    onion and cook, covered, for 7 minutes until softened, stirring occasionally.
    Add the carrot, parsnip and herbs and cook for a further 2 minutes. Remove
    the pan from the heat.
2   Meanwhile, grind the peanuts in a food processor until finely chopped then
    process the bread into crumbs. Stir into the pan with the seeds, Worcestershire
    sauce and bouillon powder. Add the beaten egg, season, and stir until combined.
3   Spoon the mixture into 2 individual greased dariole moulds. Bake for 30 minutes
    until golden and crisp on top. Turn out before serving.

21G CARBOHYDRATE PER SERVING • SERVE WITH STEAMED BROCCOLI AND
CELERIAC MASH

MAIN MEALS – VEGETARIAN

Chapter Five

Side Dishes

Whether you are looking for a vegetable accompaniment to partner a main course or an alternative to potatoes, white pasta or rice, this chapter has something for you. Some of the dishes also make an ideal light meal or snack. For lunch, you could serve the Chargrilled Thyme Courgettes with a large mixed salad, and the Spicy Chickpeas & Spinach would make a satisfying supper dish. Pulses are a combination of protein and carbohydrate and provide a nutritious range of vitamins and minerals. They are also very versatile and make the perfect creamy mash or purée, a good alternative to potatoes. The Chickpea Mash works well with many of the main meal recipes without sending the carbohydrate count off the scale. It's all too easy to ignore vegetables when restricting your carbohydrate intake but they play a vital role in a healthy, balanced diet. Some are lower in carbs than others and have a more moderate effect on blood sugar levels, hence their use in the recipes that follow. Additionally, some of the dishes have a protein element, which will help to tame the effect of the carbohydrate on blood sugar levels.

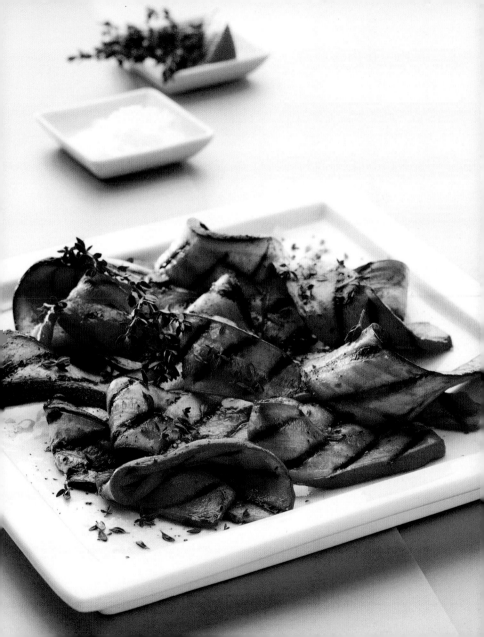

089

CHARGRILLED THYME
COURGETTES SERVES 2

sunflower oil, for brushing
2–3 courgettes/zucchini, sliced
 lengthways into fine slices

1 tsp lemon juice
1 tbsp fresh thyme
salt and freshly ground black pepper

1   Preheat the grill/broiler to medium-high and brush with oil. Arrange the
    courgettes/zucchini in a griddle pan – you may have to do this in two batches –
    and cook for 3–5 minutes, turning once, until tender but still crisp.

2   Squeeze over the lemon juice, sprinkle with thyme and season to taste.

3G CARBOHYDRATE PER SERVING

SIDE DISHES

Recipe pictured on page 125

090

CHICKPEA MASH <small>SERVES 2</small>

1 tbsp olive oil

1 clove garlic, chopped

100g/3½oz/½ cup canned chickpeas/
garbanzo beans, rinsed

2 tbsp semi-skimmed milk

salt and freshly ground black pepper

2 tbsp chopped fresh coriander/cilantro

1 Heat the oil in a saucepan and gently fry the garlic for 2 minutes, then add the chickpeas/garbanzo beans and milk and heat through for a few minutes.

2 Transfer to a blender or food processor and purée until smooth. Season to taste and stir in the fresh coriander/cilantro.

8.5G CARBOHYDRATE PER SERVING

091

SPICY CHICKPEAS & SPINACH

SERVES 2

200g/7oz/3½ cups fresh spinach leaves, tough stalks removed

1 tbsp olive oil

1 large clove garlic

1 tsp cumin seeds

85g/3oz/½ cup canned chickpeas/ garbanzo beans, rinsed

3 tbsp lemon juice

¼ tsp dried chilli flakes

salt and freshly ground black pepper

1 Wash the spinach in cold running water and place in a saucepan with nothing but the water that is already clinging onto the leaves. Cook, covered, over a medium-low heat until wilted. Drain well.

2 Meanwhile, heat the oil in a frying pan and fry the garlic, cumin and chickpeas/ garbanzo beans for 2 minutes, stirring continuously.

3 Combine the spinach and chickpea/garbanzo bean mixture in a serving bowl. Pour over the lemon juice, season well, and sprinkle with chilli flakes. Serve warm.

10G CARBOHYDRATE PER SERVING

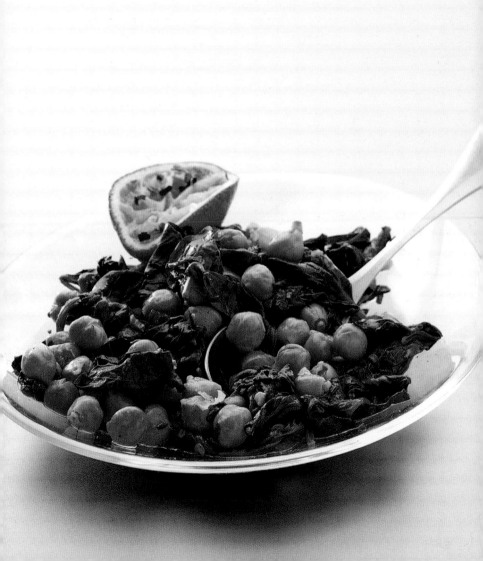

092

BRAISED LITTLE GEMS WITH CRISP BACON SERVES 2

2 slices bacon, trimmed of fat
100ml/3½fl oz/½ cup vegetable stock
 (see page 23)

10g/¼oz butter
2 Little Gem lettuces, halved lengthways
freshly ground black pepper

1   Preheat the grill/broiler to high and line a grill/broiler pan with foil. Grill/broil the
     bacon slices until crisp. Leave to cool slightly and snip into small pieces.
2   Put the stock and butter into a sauté pan and heat until the butter has melted.
     Place the lettuce halves into the pan, cover, and simmer for 2 minutes until
     softened. Remove from the pan with a slotted spoon.
3   Place the lettuces on a serving plate, scatter over the bacon pieces and season
     with pepper.

1G CARBOHYDRATE PER SERVING

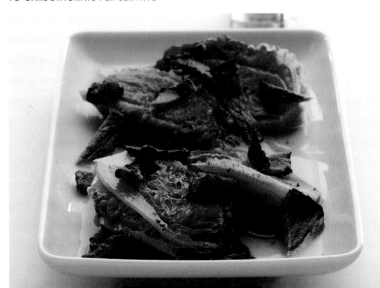

093

ARTICHOKES WITH GARLIC MAYO SERVES 2

2 artichokes

1 tsp lemon juice

salt

GARLIC MAYO:

3 tbsp reduced-fat mayonnaise

1 clove garlic, crushed

1 tsp harissa paste

1 Remove the stalks and hard outer leaves from the artichokes, then slice off the top 1cm/½in. Place stalk-end down in a saucepan of boiling salted water. Add the lemon juice and cook, half-covered, for about 20–30 minutes until an outer leaf can be pulled out easily.

2 Mix together the mayonnaise, garlic and harissa, and serve as a dip.

4G CARBOHYDRATE PER SERVING

094

SOUFFLÉ TOMATOES SERVES 3

6 vine-ripened tomatoes, tops sliced off
    and seeds scooped out
3 tbsp semi-skimmed milk
85g/3oz/¾ cup grated Gruyère cheese

1 clove garlic, crushed
2 eggs, separated
salt and freshly ground black pepper
few snipped chives, to garnish (optional)

1   Preheat the oven to 190°C/375°F/Gas 5. Lightly salt the tomatoes and place
    upside down on a plate to drain for 10 minutes.

2   Gently heat the milk in a saucepan until just warm, then add 55g/2oz/½ cup of
    the Gruyère and the garlic and egg yolks. Heat gently, stirring, until the cheese has
    melted and the mixture thickened. Remove from the heat.

3   Whisk the egg whites in a bowl until they form stiff peaks and gently fold into the
    cheese mixture using a metal spoon. Season to taste with black pepper.

4   Place the tomatoes in a lightly oiled baking pan and spoon in the soufflé mixture.
    Sprinkle with the remaining cheese and bake for 20 minutes until risen and
    golden. Sprinkle with chives and serve immediately.

6G CARBOHYDRATE PER SERVING

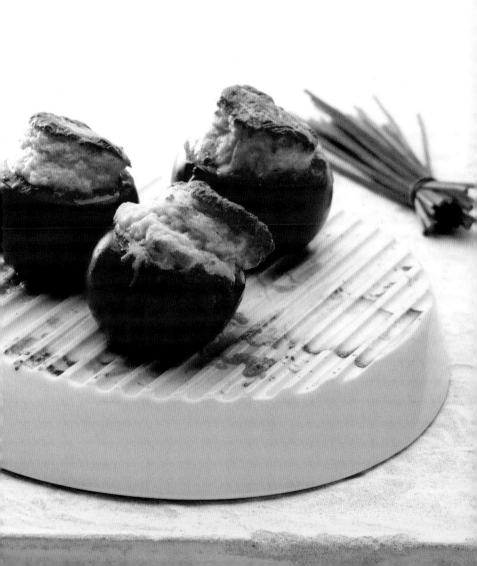

Chapter Six

Desserts

Desserts play no part in many low-carb diets. However, we all deserve the occasional treat and the following will help you have one without compromising your aims. However, although these may be lower in carbohydrates than many store-bought desserts, eating them every day is not recommended. Reserve them for special occasions or perhaps a weekend treat. Fruit is also often a no-no in some low-carb diets, especially in the restrictive induction stages, but fruit, as with vegetables, should form a part of our daily diet, providing essential fibre, vitamins and minerals, particularly antioxidants that protect us against heart disease and certain cancers. Some fruits (such as berries, melon, grapefruit and papaya) are relatively low in carbs and have a lower glycaemic index. Some of the recipes here, including Peaches with Vanilla Cream or Baked Apple with Camembert, would also make a perfect breakfast, but try to accompany them with a protein food to help tame their effect on blood sugar levels.

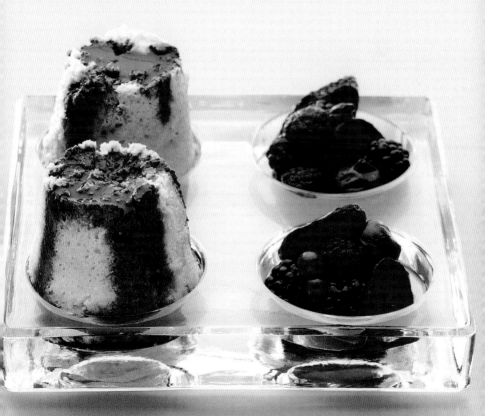

095

BAKED RICOTTA CAKES WITH BERRY SAUCE SERVES 2

sunflower oil, for greasing
140g/5oz/⅔ cup ricotta cheese
1 tbsp honey or maple syrup
½ tsp pure vanilla extract

2 egg whites
200g/7oz/1⅓ cups mixed fresh or
   frozen berries, defrosted if frozen
4 tbsp fresh apple juice

1   Preheat the oven to 180°C/350°F/Gas 4. Lightly grease 2 dariole moulds. Beat
   the ricotta, honey or syrup and vanilla extract in a bowl using a wooden spoon.

2   Whisk the egg whites until they form soft peaks. Gently fold the egg whites into
   the ricotta mixture. Spoon the mixture into the moulds. Bake for about 20 minutes
   or until risen and golden.

3   To make the berry sauce, put three-quarters of the fruit and the apple juice in
   a saucepan, then heat gently until softened. Press the fruit through a sieve to
   remove the pips.

4   Carefully remove the ricotta cakes from the moulds and place on a plate.
   Serve with the sauce and decorate with the reserved berries.

12G CARBOHYDRATE PER SERVING

Recipe pictured on page 135

096

PEACHES WITH VANILLA CREAM

SERVES 2

small knob of butter

1 tbsp fresh orange juice

2 just-ripe peaches, pitted and thickly sliced

VANILLA CREAM:

4 tbsp whipped cream

½ tsp vanilla extract

1   Mix together the whipped cream and vanilla.
2   Heat a frying pan over a medium heat. Put the butter and orange juice in the pan and heat until the butter melts. Add the peaches and cook for 2–3 minutes, turning once.
3   Arrange the peach slices in shallow bowls and pour over any juices left in the pan. Serve with a spoonful of vanilla cream.

10.5G CARBOHYDRATE PER SERVING

097

CHOCOLATE ORANGE CREAM

SERVES 2

250g/9oz/1 heaped cup ricotta
2 tbsp brandy
1 tbsp honey or maple syrup
4 tbsp fresh orange juice

1 tsp orange zest, plus fine strips,
   to decorate
20g/¾oz good-quality plain chocolate
   (70 per cent cocoa solids), finely grated

1   Beat together the ricotta, brandy, honey or syrup, orange juice and zest in a bowl.
2   Spoon a quarter of the ricotta mixture into 2 glasses and top with half the
    chocolate. Spoon the remaining ricotta mixture into the glasses and chill
    for 1 hour.
3   Before serving, sprinkle the remaining chocolate on top, then decorate with
    the orange strips.

9G CARBOHYDRATE PER SERVING

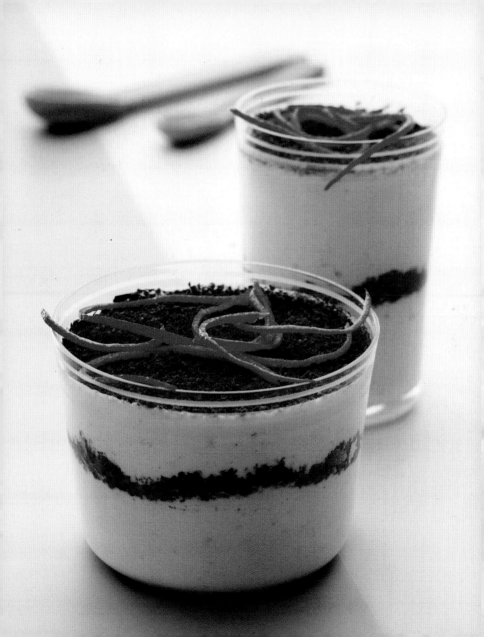

098

MANGO & LIME WITH PINEAPPLE GRANITA SERVES 2

80g/3oz/¼ cup pitted, peeled and
  cubed mango
juice of ½ lime and a few fine strips of
  lime zest, to decorate

PINEAPPLE GRANITA:
200g/7oz/1¼ cup peeled, cubed and
  cored pineapple
2 tsp grated fresh ginger

1   To make the granita, finely chop the pineapple in a food processor or blender.
2   Add the ginger, mix well, and spoon into a small freezer-proof container.
    Freeze for at least 2 hours.
3   Meanwhile, put the mango in a bowl, pour the lime juice over, stir gently, and
    chill until ready to serve.
4   Just before serving, remove the pineapple from the freezer and use a fork to
    break up the mixture into ice crystals. Divide the mango between 2 glasses or
    bowls and top with the granita. Sprinkle over the lime zest before serving.

11.5G CARBOHYDRATE PER SERVING

099

BAKED APPLE WITH CAMEMBERT SERVES 2

1 dessert apple, halved vertically
and cored

2 tbsp dry white wine

55g/2oz Camembert, sliced and with
rind cut off

1 Preheat the oven to 190°C/375°F/Gas 5. Arrange the 2 apple halves on a large
   piece of foil and spoon the wine over. Fold up the foil to make a parcel and place
   in a roasting pan.

2 Bake the apple for 15–20 minutes until tender.

3 Preheat the grill/broiler to medium and line the grill/broiler pan with foil.

4 Remove the apples from their parcel and place the Camembert slices on top.
   Grill/broil for about 3 minutes until the cheese has melted.

8.5G CARBOHYDRATE PER SERVING

100

CUSTARD VANILLA CREAM SERVES 1

1 tbsp flaked almonds

1 tbsp sunflower seeds

100ml/3½fl oz/½ cup thick natural
 bio yogurt

1 egg yolk

½ tsp pure vanilla extract

55g/2oz/⅓ cup raspberries, hulled

1   Lightly toast the almonds and sunflower seeds in a dry frying pan until golden.

2   Put the yogurt and egg yolk in a heavy saucepan. Heat gently, stirring frequently,
    until the mixture begins to bubble.

3   Add the vanilla extract and stir gently until the mixture thickens to the consistency
    of custard.

4   Divide the raspberries between 2 glasses. Spoon in the custard and serve sprinkled
    with the almonds and seeds.

7G CARBOHYDRATE PER SERVING

INDEX OF RECIPE NAMES

The numbers below refer to pages, not recipe numbers.

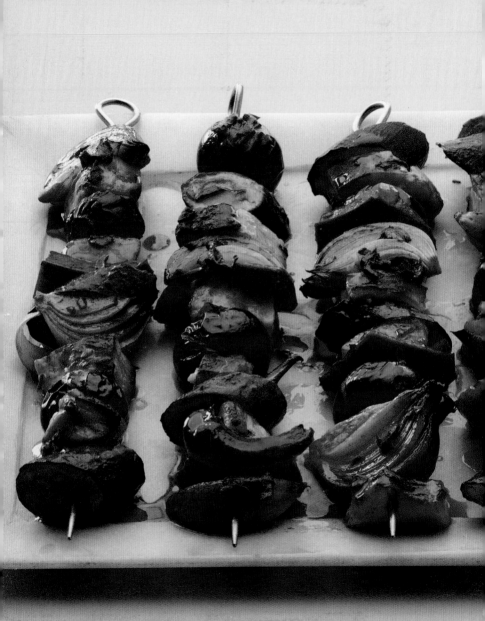